FLAT

FLAT

RECLAIMING MY BODY FROM BREAST CANCER

CATHERINE GUTHRIE

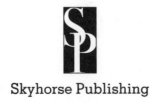

Skyhorse Publishing

Skyhorse Publishing books may be purchased in bulk at special discounts for sales promotion, corporate gifts, fund-raising, or educational purposes. Special editions can also be created to specifications. For details, contact the Special Sales Department, Skyhorse Publishing, 307 West 36th Street, 11th Floor, New York, NY 10018 or info@skyhorsepublishing.com.

Skyhorse® and Skyhorse Publishing® are registered trademarks of Skyhorse Publishing, Inc.®, a Delaware corporation.

Visit our website at www.skyhorsepublishing.com.

10 9 8 7 6 5 4 3 2 1

Library of Congress Cataloging-in-Publication Data is available on file.

Cover design by Jenny Zemanek
Cover illustration: iStockphoto

Print ISBN: 978-1-5107-3291-9
Ebook ISBN: 978-1-5107-3294-0

Printed in the United States of America

For Mary

CHAPTER 1

The lump appeared in January 2009.

Correction—it didn't appear so much as reveal itself.

I was alone in bed. A place I'd always felt safe or, more accurately, at home. It still rankles me that the lump found me there.

But I'm getting ahead of myself. On that cold Sunday morning, I was alone in a tangle of bedsheets that still held the heat of two bodies. Sounds of morning filtered up through the heating vents. The rhythmic clank of the dog's tags against her metal bowl, the murmurings of NPR hosts, the click-click-click of the gas stove's ignition. Amid this serenade, I stretched and lolled. With a yawn, I rolled onto my stomach.

Ouch!

My breast felt bruised. My fingers prodded the area, taking their job seriously. With determined tenderness, they tried to reproduce the sharpness of the pain but found nothing of note. They did, however, find a tender spot, the size of a nickel, above my left breast. Near the sore spot was a small mole. As innocent as a freckle. As familiar as a signpost. No bigger than a lentil. That mole was flat, not raised. A perfectly round dot. The mole had been there for as long as I could remember. Or had it?

A few minutes later, in the shower, beneath a drumbeat of water, my fingers returned to the tender spot, like bloodhounds circling a scent. Yes, there it was. My brain sketched a quick story about how the seam of my bra had irritated the mole, causing the soreness. In hindsight, that was ridiculous. I'd had the bra for ages, and the tender spot was not on the mole so much as in the proximity of it. But, when faced with trouble, the mind is a nimble storyteller.

And then I felt it—a protrusion the size of a pebble.

My reaction was on par with my personality. Outwardly calm but inwardly freaking the fuck out. When in doubt, go through the motions. Pumping more bath gel onto the washcloth, I ran it over my arms and legs. I squeezed conditioner into my palm and worked it through my close-cropped hair. Adrenaline cracked and popped through my veins like a cheap string of firecrackers.

I knew a thing or two about breast lumps. I was a magazine journalist, and women's health was my specialty. Writing about breast cancer was my bread and butter: how to prevent it, how to detect it, how to survive it, how to talk to your best friend about it. Risk factors, statistics, and treatment options rattled off my tongue at the slightest provocation. Over the years, survivors had taken me into their confidence. Breast cancer surgeons had walked me through evolutions in the field—how the standard of care had transitioned from mastectomies to lumpectomies, cancer carved from a breast, like a worm from an apple. On the subject of breast lumps, I also had firsthand experience: a benign lump in my right breast. The harmless fibroadenoma had arrived in my late twenties, its discovery and diagnosis triggering an avalanche of twenty-something angst. Was this new lump the thirty-something sequel?

Out of the shower, onto the white bathmat. I cinched the towel around my waist. Rivulets of water ran down my legs as my fingers re-familiarized themselves with the fibroadenoma. Then, they moved to the lump in the opposite breast. Back and forth. Compare and contrast. My eyes squeezed shut, as if to amplify the transmission of information from my fingertips, crowded as they were with touch receptors.

The new lump was everything the old lump was not. Solid, unyielding, jagged, a broken tooth. Against the tips of my fingers, the benign lump was rubbery, slippery, friendly. My knees wobbled. I sat down hard on the lid of the toilet. Stark winter sunlight glinted off the bathroom's high-gloss subway tiles and silvery chrome fixtures. A year ago, we'd remodeled. It was our first home-improvement project, our first real effort to turn the downtrodden house into a home. We'd chosen glossy white tiles and polished fixtures because they were bright and clean, but now they only felt cold and sterile.

Downstairs, Mary stood at the stove holding a slotted spoon, her eyes fixed on a simmering pot of water. With the exception of poached eggs, the woman cooked everything on high heat for maximum efficiency. The higher the flame, the faster the cook time. The faster the cook time, the sooner she could get back to work. Most days I was surprised she ate anything at all.

I dressed, padded downstairs, sidled up to her.

"Somebody needs a hug," I said, using a line we'd cribbed from a TV show.

"I want one of those," she responded on cue.

She lowered the spoon and opened her arms. I snuggled into the warm crook of her neck and the soft folds of her plush bathrobe. The sweet smells of clean laundry and morning musk muffled the firecrackers.

What if I said nothing?

Silence was my go-to strategy. Here's one way this could go: two weeks from now, we'd be sitting at the breakfast table. I'd tell her I'd had a scare and gone to the doctor. Dr. F had checked it out and said "not to worry." Just another fibroadenoma. Mary would be hurt, but she'd get over it because I would be okay.

But, no. Our relationship had issues, but secrecy wasn't one of them.

"What up, nut-nut?"

"I found a lump."

"Where?"

She stepped back. Put her hands on my shoulders, slid them down to my elbows. Her eyes roamed my clothes, as if she could see through them with X-ray vision.

"My boob."

"Let me feel?"

My left hand pulled the neckline of my shirt aside, while my right guided her hand to my chest, placing her fingers on the tender spot near the mole.

Her face clouded.

"Call the doctor?"

"I will."

And just like that she swiveled back to the stove. A flip of her wrist snuffed the burner, the spoon rescued the egg and slid it onto a piece of toast. Mary was a social scientist and a researcher. She liked facts. The lump was merely a starting point for investigation, no quantifiable data yet. Mary refused to traffic in fear. Me? I turned into Chicken Little at the slightest whiff of worry. When that happened, my clucking sent Mary deep into Mr. Rogers territory. The more I squawked, the calmer and more sing-song-y she got.

"I'm sure it's nothing," she said, taking her breakfast to the table.

"Yeah. You're probably right."

I poured a cup of coffee and tried to relax, but the din of my body's alarm was not easily silenced. She didn't know as much as I did about breast lumps. My fibroadenoma scare had happened in 1997, the year before we met. She wasn't as familiar with the friendly, rubbery contours of my benign lump. She hadn't been at my side when the doctor had told twenty-six-year-old me that cancerous lumps feel jagged, stuck in place, like a tick dug into the side of a dog. That's the kind of vivid detail an anxiety-prone health journalist doesn't forget.

Much of this story takes place in Bloomington, Indiana, a small city of 85,000 in the middle of nowhere. Go to the middle of the country, zoom out, and picture the face of a clock with Chicago at 12 o'clock and Nashville at 6. Locate St. Louis at 9 o'clock and Columbus, Ohio, at 3. Then draw a line from each of these four cities until they meet in the middle of the clock face. That center point is Indianapolis. Now slide your eyes southwest across fifty miles of farmland. Now you've found Bloomington.

I wouldn't have known where Bloomington was, either, except that it hugs the main campus of Indiana University, Mary's employer. Worth knowing, too, is that the University props up the city's economy, creating an artificial bubble of prosperity. Home prices are among the highest in the state, and dollars spent by faculty, staff, and students buoy local businesses and give the town a wholesome sheen. An island of homogeneity, Bloomington is a safe place for parents to park their offspring for four years. And, on any given day, campus is a sea of twiggy girls in UGGs and slothful boys with artfully tousled hair.

Don't get me wrong. Bloomington oozes curb appeal. It is the quintessential all-American college town. The kind of Truman-show-esque city that tops lists of the ten most scenic college campuses and best places for retirees. At its heart is a proud courthouse built from limestone mined from quarries just outside of town. Surrounding the courthouse is a solid wall of local businesses: the Scholars Inn Bakehouse, Indiana Running Company, and Goods for Cooks. Mom-and-pop shops are squeezed shoulder-to-shoulder around the square, a fortress against corporatization, cherished by students, staff, and faculty. Other local businesses seem to survive on the power of nostalgia alone, like the Caveat Emptor, a cavernous used bookstore with claustrophobic shelves, floor-to-ceiling stacks, and air thick with book mold.

And you haven't even seen the campus yet. From the courthouse, turn east on Kirkwood Street and saunter past the coffee houses, farm-to-table restaurants, and vintage-clothing stores. In less than ten minutes, you'll see two stone pillars, the Sample Gates, framing the school's west boundary. If you were to ask me, this is the prettiest entrance to the campus. Look past the gates to the wide, welcoming pedestrian path and views of ivy-covered buildings. I'd visited the campus twice before, and it was this entrance I conjured when Mary accepted her first tenure-track teaching job in 2004, and it was this small Midwestern city that we tucked ourselves into for the ride.

But back to the lump. Two days after it asserted itself, I pointed the nose of our green Subaru (what else?) toward the internist's office on the west side of town. Dr. F practiced in a red brick building shimmed into a bland office park. This was Bloomington's not-so-charming side, the grease-clogged engine under the city's shiny hood. Local landmarks were the only way to find my doctor's nondescript building. Go past the White River Co-Op, a farm-supply store where the TV was always tuned to Fox News. Turn left at the local Buffalo Wild Wings franchise, where cheap beer and flat-screen televisions lured frat boys on weekends. Go right at Williams Brothers Pharmacy, the last locally owned drug store in town, and you've arrived.

I left the car unlocked, figuring it would be a quick in-and-out visit. I'd gotten an annual checkup less than three months ago. My girls got the all clear that day, so surely the lump was nothing. Right? Surely this was just my Chicken Little talking. Mary and I both knew I could be a bit of a hypochondriac. We wrote it off as an occupational hazard.

A few minutes later, inside the exam room, my sock-clad heels tapped against the steel base of the table while my eyes roved the walls for distraction. The decor consisted of an illustrated guide to a self-breast exam, a flyer for a domestic violence hotline, and a clear plastic magazine rack sprouting rumpled issues of *Ladies' Home Journal* and *Fitness*. I'd written for both and been disappointed by my editors' edicts that health stories should have weight-loss angles and contain no words with more than two syllables.

Editors of women's magazines often assume their readers prefer cotton candy to serious journalism. I longed to write meaty, thought-provoking articles like those that filled the feature wells of magazines, such as *Harper's* and the *Atlantic.* Stories with political and cultural gravitas. But most women's magazines insisted on talking down to their readers, assigning only chatty, service-y pieces. Articles that offered quick takeaways about how to be a better wife, mother, daughter, or best friend. Why did I keep at it? Because someday I'd be better positioned to place smart, interesting stories that would make a difference in women's lives. Maybe I'd influence someone's health decisions for the better. In hindsight, however, I was playing it safe. After a lifetime of wanting to assimilate into the world of straight women, writing for them gave me a sense of confidence. Maybe my bookish, queer-self had something to offer straight women after all.

Knuckles rapped on the door and Dr. F bustled into the room cradling a laptop. She and I were both in our late thirties, but she looked older, more maternal. Maybe it was our style. Oversized sweaters and ripped jeans pegged me as someone stuck in a '90s-grunge phase. She had a penchant for prairie skirts and floral-print blouses, a Laura-Ingalls vibe that I found both comforting and mildly alarming, as if the clothes might reflect the medicine she practiced. She settled the computer on the room's pint-sized countertop and squinted at the screen. After a few pecks at the keyboard, she peered up at me through her oval glasses.

"So, what's up?"

"Oh, just a lump." Maybe if I adopted a casual tone, the lump wouldn't be a big deal.

She nodded. "Let's check it out."

A yellowed poster of a waterfall was taped to the white ceiling tiles. Dr. F creased back the paper gown and settled her cool, dry fingers on the edge of my breast—starting at the outer perimeter and working toward the nipple. Slow. Deliberate. Her concentric circles tightened. The way her fingers mashed my breast reminded me of my mother's handling of raw pie dough.

Early on the morning of a holiday or a family occasion, my mother would retrieve the refrigerated balls of flour, water, and lard she'd prepared the night before, sprinkle flour on the laminate countertop, and roll out the stiff pastry until it was a quarter-inch thick, rotating the angle of the rolling pin with each pass. Then, she'd drape the delicate blanket over an aluminum pie pan, ease it into the bottom, and use the pads of her fingers to press the dough flat and even.

Dr. F reached my nipple and came up empty. Nothing. She hadn't felt it. Her thin lips pressed into a straight line. She lifted her hands, paused, took a centering breath. She returned to the start.

As her fingers smoothed and pressed my body's compliant flesh, a voice in my head began to root for her.

A little to the left.

Press harder.

You've almost got it.

Some part of me wanted her to find it. Wanted her to feel successful, yes, but also wanted to trust her skill, her knowledge. She was the doctor after all.

Her fingertips went round and round, like water circling a drain.

Gaaah! What was the matter with me? Why was I turning my scary breast-lump appointment into a diagnostic win for her?

My elbows pressed into the exam table as I sat up. The tissue paper under my ass ripped.

"Here. The lump is easier to feel when I'm sitting."

She took my bossiness in stride.

"The lump is at six o'clock." An edge of impatience was creeping into my voice. "See that mole?"

The flat lentil-like shape was coming in handy.

"Yeah, that's it. Okay. Now, go down an inch."

Touchdown. Her fingertips landed on the lump.

They paused, then lightly tiptoed across its surface. Up and down. Side to side. The shard of glass gave up nothing. Did her brain tick through the list of traits separating a benign lump from a malignant one? Hard versus soft? Pliable versus static? If so, she didn't show it. Her expression was neither surprised nor concerned.

Her head shook. "You're too young for breast cancer, but I'll order a mammogram, just in case."

And with that she spun to the sink to wash her hands. As a family practitioner, her job was to handle the minor stuff, like ear infections, chicken pox, and strep throat. More serious cases were passed up the chain of command. But I didn't want to graduate. I wanted her to say, *you're fine, nothing to worry about, and see ya next year.*

Instead she said, "My nurse will stop by with more information." And she was gone. In the click of the door's latch, I heard, "You are no longer my responsibility."

As a patient, it is easy to feel dismissed by the harmless gestures of medical professionals. Exchanges that were fraught for me were routine for them. They couldn't possibly put themselves in the shoes of every patient. But, oh, how different things would be if they did.

I pulled on my gray long-sleeve thermal and black wool sweater, grabbed my Timbuk2 messenger bag, and cracked the door open. I gophered my head out. The hall was empty. Did she tell me to stay put?

Then her nurse appeared and held out a business card for the Southern Indiana Radiological Services. She'd called and made me an appointment. Pinpricks needled the back of my neck. Nothing made me more nervous than expedited medical care.

The car slid home on glazed streets. I cursed under my breath as the back wheels fishtailed through a four-way stop. Mary had offered to drive me to the appointment, and I'd said no. Unlike me, she loved winter driving, a skill she'd mastered living seasonally near Lake Tahoe before we met. "They didn't call me Mary-o-Andretti for nothing," she bragged every winter as she steered with steady confidence through ice, sleet, and snow. My insistence on self-reliance would imperil our relationship, but I didn't know this yet. I couldn't see that Mary's chivalrous gestures were her way of seeking connection. I saw them only as a judgment of my ability to fend for myself. The more she offered to help, the more independent I wanted to be.

Steering into the driveway, the car lumbered over a snow bank and into its parking spot. With a quick twist of the key, I cut the engine, and silence fell like a weighted curtain. My eyelids lowered as a paralysis worked its way down my body. Maybe just a little car nap. But my health-writer brain insisted on popping the lid off its worry box and holding facts and percentages up to the light like glass baubles.

Annual number of women in the US who die of breast cancer: 41,000

Annual number of women who are diagnosed with the disease: 236,000

Number of breast cancer patients who are younger than forty: 6.6 percent

Number of Americans living with breast cancer who don't know they are ill: upwards of a million

This wasn't helping!

Go inside, go upstairs, get to work.

My mammogram was scheduled for February 2—two weeks away. Simple, purposeful goals were good. Deadlines would distract me.

At the sound of my key in the lock, Emma began to bark from inside the house. Barking was her favorite pastime, and her body was built for volume. She was a barrel-chested boxer-mix we'd adopted at eight weeks from West Virginia Boxer Rescue. We were drawn to her independent and impish personality. As a puppy, she'd been cautious and curious. But she'd grown into an alpha girl who patrolled our home's periphery like it was the Korean DMZ. Marching from room to room and window to window, resting her whiskery chin on each sill, and perking her ears, she scanned the sidewalk for evildoers, such as children waiting for the school bus. If anyone broached her territory, she'd give 'em the business. But her posturing was mostly show. She greeted people by wagging not just her stub tail but also curving her body back and forth, a move we'd dubbed her "full body wag."

She came bounding down the stairs as I opened the side door, not stopping until she was leaning against my legs and air-licking my face. The flat of my palm made a deep, hollow sound as it thumped her side. My momentum for work slid off my shoulders as easily as my winter coat. Deadlines could wait. Brushing the dog hair from my jeans, I grabbed the remote and surrendered to the brown couch. Barack Obama was being sworn into his first term in office. Maybe I could still catch some of the coverage.

Before I move on, the brown couch is more than a minor character in this story. So, a full introduction is fitting.

The brown couch was L-shaped, and it floated in the middle of our living room, like a life raft. Because we had a large dog, we'd chosen an upholstery the color of dried mud. Previously, Emma abided by our rule that dogs weren't allowed to jump on the furniture unless invited, but the minute the brown couch arrived, she laid claim to the L's short outcropping. In turn, Mary had dibs on the bottom corner of the "L." That meant the length of the brown couch, the "L's" long arm, was all mine. Because my back tired easily, aching by the end of the day, I was often horizontal on the brown couch, my feet nudging their way into Mary's lap where she would rub them—vigorously and then absentmindedly—as we watched TV. Bookending the brown couch were spindly floor lamps. And underneath the couch, a multi-colored, braided wool rug served as a garish lily pad. From your seat on the couch, you could gaze to the right, out the windows and through the negligible front yard, and notice people and cars passing by. In the middle of the room, equidistant between the front and side doors, the brown couch expressed a twinge of vulnerability. Its occupant could never fully relax. But I'll speak for myself. For all

I know, Mary never gave the frigging couch a second thought. We were different that way.

In the living room, the brown couch faced both our fireplace and the TV. Because we often worked from home, we had a strict "no television during the day" policy, though we made exceptions for breaking news. Today, I could use Obama's inauguration to justify a couple of hours of couch time. Emma hopped up, made three circles, and harrumphed herself into a ball. I flipped channels through a succession of talking heads. Still shots of the White House filled the background. Damn. I'd missed the ceremony's pomp and circumstance: the oath, the hand on the Bible, the inaugural poem, the rituals of democracy that reassured me of America's civility and sanity. I was still channel surfing when the phone rang.

The caller ID flashed. Guilt tugged at my chest like a fishing line. Shit. That girl forgot nothing. My sister Beth was the only person aside from Mary who knew about the lump and the appointment.

The youngest of my three siblings, Beth had a big heart and a tongue sharpened on the family stone. I was five years older, but we'd forged an early bond. First, through my little-girl desire to mother someone and later, through our shared coping mechanisms of sarcasm and snark. As adolescents, she was the champion eye-roller and I was the put-down queen.

My family was a Tootsie Pop, layer upon layer of hard feelings (resentment, cynicism, sarcasm) wrapped around a soft, sweet center. Everyone wanted to be loved but no one agreed on the terms. To my father, love looked like being a reliable provider. To my mother, love meant sacrifice. To me, love felt like being seen not just for who I was but for who I was trying to be.

Beth was the first person in my family who saw me. As adults we shared the same immature sense of humor. We emoted first and thought second. We each fell in love with a person kinder than ourselves in hopes that it would rub off.

Eight short weeks ago, Beth and her husband had had their first child, a daughter Caroline. I'd been at the birth, held Beth's hand during labor, and performed a goofy dance as I changed the baby's first poopy diaper. Now Beth was home on maternity leave and our chats were timed to her breastfeeding cycle. When Caroline latched on, Beth dialed my number.

I answered the phone.

"Hey, just calling to find out how it went." Her tone was light and upbeat. Motherhood sounded good on her.

"Oh, well, the doctor felt it. It's a lump alright."

"Yeah, sooooooo, what comes next?" The baby snuffled and grunted. My fingernails strummed at the rubbery buttons on the TV remote. Picture Beth in a new construction townhome in the suburbs of Washington, DC, late-afternoon light bathing her high-ceilinged living room. She sits in a plush chair-and-a-half, a green polka-dotted nursing pillow around her waist, a chubby baby in her lap. Her husband is on his way home from his nine-to-five government job.

"I need a mammogram but there is only one place to go in Bloomington, and the soonest I can get in is next month," I said, shivering under a thin blanket on the brown couch. The dark red walls of our living room canceling the sun. A chill seeped through the horsehair plaster walls. I dug my toes under the weight of the sleeping dog, wicking her warmth. Mary wouldn't be home for at least two more hours, maybe longer.

"You know, Indianapolis isn't that far from Bloomington," Beth said. "It's a big city, I bet it has lots of places you could get a mammogram without the long wait."

"Yeah, I know." Impatience serrated my voice. It bugged me when people played Mr. Fix-it with my problems. Peppering me with reasonable solutions. The tone in my voice would have been enough to discourage most people from continuing the conversation, but not Beth. "So, do you want me to look up some places?" Static filled my ear. This was the sound of her dropping the phone while switching Caroline to the other breast. Then she was back. "So, what's it gonna be?"

"No. I got it," I said, shoving the blanket off my lap. Could she hear my eyes roll? "I'll call you later."

A few minutes later, a quick search for "mammogram + Indianapolis" brought up several possibilities, and, in less than thirty minutes, I'd cut my wait time in half. My new appointment was at St. Vincent Breast Center in Indianapolis the following Monday—six days away.

CHAPTER 2

Early on the morning of the mammogram, Mary's fingers grazed the black knobs of the Forester's meager dashboard like talismans, adjusting the blower, dialing up the radio, and punching the button for the back window defrost. My hands burrowed deep into the pockets of my down winter coat as she drove past the darkened storefronts of pizza joints, bars, and tattoo parlors—the economic lifeblood of a college town.

Mary had offered to drive me to St. Vincent Hospital in Carmel, Indiana, a suburb north of Indianapolis, and this time I'd said yes even though we both feared she couldn't afford to take time off. Like most assistant professors, she worked up to eighty hours a week. Mornings were for class prep and teaching, afternoons disappeared into a whirl of office hours and committee meetings, evenings went to email, and weekends were swallowed by grading. "It won't always be like this," she assured me. "After tenure is when life begins."

The tenure process would take six years, what felt like an eternity, but whenever I chafed at the demands of her university job she reminded me of its many perks. Namely, health benefits. In the past, with incomes quilted from grants and freelance-writing gigs, we'd gotten by with decent-enough coverage. Mary had graduate student health insurance through her program at the University of California, San Diego, and I had a catastrophic policy for freelancers. But, as we edged into our thirties, we knew we were rolling the dice. A serious accident or life-threatening illness would have bankrupted us and potentially our parents, too. When we found out her job offer at Indiana came with health insurance for both of us, we were surprised. Domestic partnership benefits were rare in the Midwest in 2004, even at universities, but beneficent policies attracted better talent. For weeks after she'd accepted the job, we beamed with our good fortune. Everything from here on out would be gravy.

From the passenger seat, I studied the downturned corners of Mary's mouth, the colorlessness of her winter-white cheeks, the deep vertical line between her eyebrows. "A byproduct of all that thinking," I'd say when she'd fret about it. But, in bed at night, when she'd drop to sleep—Mary dropped, never drifted—and her head lay heavy on my shoulder, my left hand held my current library book while my right arm held her close, my fingers drifting to the line, massaging it in hopes of easing the worries beneath.

But in the car that morning, the mood was crashing fast. Absurdity was in order. I piped up, "So, I read an article in one of my women's magazines about how novel experiences breathe new life into a relationship."

She nodded, her eyes flicking to the rearview mirror and back to the highway.

"Maybe exploring medical facilities in the outskirts of Indianapolis will be a turn on."

Mary grinned and crooned, "Oooooh yeah, baby. Take me to Carmel or lose me forever."

No matter how flat my jokes fell, Mary would always pick them up, sharpen them, and toss them back in unexpected ways that loosened up my serious side. When she wasn't stressed out about work, she was one of the most magnetic people I'd ever met. Her gaze a spotlight. When turned on you, everything else dimmed.

Mary liked to say she'd "never met a stranger," and I believed her. A cultural anthropologist, she was genuinely curious about what made people tick and how they saw the world. She charmed everyone, from the provost of the University to the waitress at our favorite Bloomington greasy spoon, Wee Willie's. But charm wasn't the right word. Charm suggests ulterior motive, like a politician vying for votes, and Mary had none. She embraced everyone and every new adventure with a deep well of optimism fed by her trust in people's innate goodness. Like most couples, we balanced one another. On good days, my pragmatism clarified and grounded her larger-than-life ambitions and utopian ideals. On bad days, my anxiety-prone, safety-first attitude obliterated her spontaneity.

At St. Vincent, we clomped through the mammography center's waiting room in our toboggans, gloves, and puffy jackets. Startled couples looked up and settled back into their nests of coats and bags like mating pairs of birds. Between each twosome sat a glass end table with fanned magazines—*Sports Illustrated* for him and *InStyle* for her. How I envied straight couples at times like these. A man and wife side by side, weathering the threat of illness together, 'til death do us part.

As two women, we lack clarity. Mary and I were often mistaken for sisters or friends. Having to explain our relationship at moments when I was nervous or stressed was taxing at best, humiliating at worst. And the queer community's god-awful, agreed-upon lexicon for same-sex relationships didn't help the situation.

"She's my partner," I'd say.

Oh, really? What business are you in?

"I mean my domestic partner."

Hmm . . . so is that a home-decorating business?

"No, I mean she is my spouse."

"Oh, so you're married?"

Well, no, that's illegal in Indiana.

"Really? That's not legal here? Are you sure? I could have sworn gay marriage was a thing now."

"Um . . . yeah . . . no."

Exasperated, I'd reduce the most significant person in my life to a pronoun. "Can she come with me?" and "Is it okay if she stays?"

I signed in while Mary made a beeline for two open chairs. She dug deep into her canvas backpack. Thwump! A stack of student papers landed on her lap.

I sank into the seat next to her and stared at my lap. My fingertips pried at the tip of a feather poking through a seam in my coat. Ideally, I would have told her about my anxiety. Asked her to put away her grading and sit with me, even if it meant staring at the wall together. Maybe even hold my hand. But the invisible line of connection between us—the current that carried the sharpened jokes, the shared vocabulary, and the nuanced looks—had gone slack. How to tighten it without seeming needy? Neediness was Mary's kryptonite. I picked at the feather in my coat until it slid out of the pinhole in the fabric, twirled it between my fingers, watched as it floated to the floor.

A nurse threw open the door and launched my name into the room. "Guthrie!"

The nesting couples all looked up in unison.

Mary clambered to collect her things, while I gestured toward the nurse to ask if it was okay that we both follow her.

She tapped her foot and jabbed her chin at Mary. "Yep. It's okay. Your friend can come, too."

The next waiting room was quiet and dim with black leather couches, a flat-screen TV turned to CNN, and a stack of golf magazines. Unfazed by being the only woman in the room, Mary broke for the couch but not before touching my arm. Her hazel eyes, warm and relaxed, said, "Hey, you got this."

The nurse pointed me to the patients' dressing room. Inside were two sinks, a large mirror, and a half dozen lockers. On the countertop was an assortment of toiletries: Kleenex, unscented baby wipes, and a generic can of aerosol deodorant. I gave myself a self-congratulatory pat on the back. Because I was only thirty-eight, I'd never had a mammogram, but I'd written articles on the dos and don'ts. Knowing many deodorants contain trace minerals that look suspicious on film, I'd gone without deodorant that morning. I'd even thought to slip a travel-sized roll-on into my bag to apply afterward. I was already plotting the pitch to my editor at *Health Magazine*—"A Breast Lump How-to Guide: Getting Through a False Alarm."

Ten minutes later, in a room down the hall, a young woman with freckles and minty breath shoved my left breast into the mammography machine. The machine was bigger than I'd anticipated, the steel colder. Reframing this experience as first-person research for a future article settled my nerves. As she adjusted the plates for multiple angles, my discomfort drew out my awkward sense of humor. Chances are I made at least one bad joke about being a mammogram virgin, but all I remember for sure was her patient smile as the machine's glass plates pancaked my breast.

An ultrasound was next. I lay down on the metal gurney. The radiation technician peeled back the left side of my hospital gown, squeezed cold, clear gel on my breast, picked up a Mr. Microphone, and slid it back and forth, smearing the goo across my chest. Craning my neck, I could just see the laptop-sized screen. The technician offered a quick tutorial using her free hand as a pointer. She explained that the undulating horizontal lines at the bottom of the screen were stratifications of muscle and the wispy-looking formations closer to the top were layers of fat and skin. If I squinted, the image was a black-and-white beach scene, with long horizontal lines of deeply hued water under thin, cottony clouds.

The microphone stopped moving. "There it is," she said.

I strained for a closer look.

"There," she said pointing.

"That?"

"Yes."

Her finger rested near a small round cloud floating among the sky's long, thin ones. An ominous sign in an otherwise serene seascape. She zoomed in to take its measurement: 1.37 centimeters. Then, using quick-key commands, she snapped pictures from various angles.

"We'll need to have a radiologist take a look. You may need a biopsy."

She wiped the gel off my breast.

"How long will that take?"

She glanced at the clock.

"How long are you willing to wait?"

"As long as it takes." A thickness formed in the back of my throat. Mary had hoped to get back for a department meeting. Now I'd sentenced us both to a day of waiting.

"I'll see what I can do."

Thirty minutes later, Mary and I were parked at a Burger King up the street with veggie burgers in our laps and a bag of fries balanced on the gearshift. In times of stress, the women in my family reached for fat and sugar.

With four small children, my mother had little choice but to resort to food bribes. All tantrum-free trips to the doctor ended at Plehn's Bakery, an institution in Louisville, Kentucky. The minute my siblings and I scooted off the backseat of my mother's wood-paneled station wagon and onto the sidewalk next to Plehn's, our noses lifted to the sweet scent of baked goods. The kitchen's exhaust fans were strategically placed to sweep passersby into the shop on the combined scent of sugar and butter, a culinary magic carpet ride. Inside, bells on the bakery door jingled. A number dispenser stuck out its tongue and told us to get in line. While we waited, my eyes ate everything in sight. Against the left-hand wall was an old-fashioned soda fountain with four padded stools that wobbled and spun. Above the counter was a black-and-white pegboard menu listing sandwich offerings, such as pimento cheese, benedictine, and country ham—three staples of every Guthrie family birthday, holiday get-together, and (of course) Derby party. Along the other walls stood gleaming pastry cases filled with chocolate eclairs, jelly donuts, elaborately decorated gingerbread men, iced sugar cookies, petite fours, and dolly buns.

Floating behind the cases were dew-faced girls from Sacred Heart, the Catholic all-girl's high school down the street. My mother had grown up in the neighborhood and attended Sacred Heart, just as my father had gone to the neighboring all-boys version, Trinity. My grandmother kept a running tab at the bakery for sixty-odd years. Louisville was that kind of town. Growing up, I'd idolized the graceful, all-powerful bakery goddesses at Plehn's. Their beatific smiles, their ability to squeeze a dozen fruit-filled breakfast pastries into a white, waxed box without any jostling or smearing. Their dexterity in quickly crisscrossing all four sides of the box with white kitchen string, only to cinch it tight and tie it off with a perfect bow.

Back in the car, my stomach growled at the salty, greasy, smell of French fries. The burger's foil wrapper crinkled and caught droplets of mayonnaise and strands of wilted lettuce before they could land on my jeans. Mary's hand disappeared into the bag of fries.

"So, how do you think this morning went?" she asked.

"Not great." I pulled a shred of brown lettuce out of my burger and wiped it on my napkin.

"Anything in particular?"

"I dunno. Just a feeling."

"If only you had a ticker tape running across your forehead to tell me what you were thinking."

I nodded, but we both knew that wasn't my way, it was hers.

Mary's thoughts sprung from her lips fully formed. She was a linear thinker and a gifted debater. In thirty seconds, she could construct a rock-solid argument for or against any topic. My thoughts meandered. Percolated. Aged. Often, I wrote first and spoke second. For me, speaking was the culmination of extensive thought. For Mary, speaking and thinking happened at the same time. Talking was how she processed information.

Back at St. Vincent's, the motions of that morning were repeated. Waiting room. Dressing room. Exam room. Soon, I would find the predictability of such rituals reassuring, but for now, things still felt novel.

By 3 p.m., I was lying on the exam table, a blue smock covering my chest, when the radiologist loped through the door. She had a long face, framed by two curtains of dark brown hair. After introducing herself, she assessed the readiness of the room and adjusted the machine to her liking.

"This won't hurt, just a small prick to numb the area," she said. Her lanky frame looked even longer in the standard-issue doctor's whites.

"Sure, that's what they all say," I riffed.

"Have you had a needle biopsy before?"

It had been ten years since my fibroadenoma scare led to my first and only needle biopsy.

"Yes." False confidence streaked my voice.

"So you know the drill."

Using the ultrasound wand, she located the lump as the technician had done earlier, but instead of taking pictures she grabbed a metal, gun-shaped tool from the instrument tray.

Clack! The needle burned as it sunk into my flesh.

With the force of the jab, the needle drew a thin tissue sample, the width of angel hair pasta, into its hollow shaft. Several more samples were needed to boost the test's accuracy.

"You're not the right age for this," she said, frowning at the screen. "It's probably nothing."

Clack! Clack! Clack!

I fought the urge to yank away from the cold jabs of the metal, its sound and pressure like a cap gun.

Finally, a pause. "I think we've got enough," she said. "Just one more thing."

She fitted another small tube into the needle's chamber and squinted at the screen. Her finger pressed the trigger and the metal barrel jolted against my breast. She nodded and pointed to the screen. In the sky, next to the rain cloud, was a stark white object.

"It's a metal tag. It stays in place and shows up on future mammo-grams to let doctors know we biopsied this lump."

The tag was a UFO, bright and white and lodged between the waves of my body's seascape. The tag's sharp boundaries were crisp and clean, irrefutable evidence that the lump had been discovered, claimed, and biopsied by a medical professional.

"So I've been tagged and released," I joked, thinking of how I'd taken Emma to the vet for a microchip last summer. How I'd held her head as the technician's needle sunk the rice-grain-sized metal tag into her scruff.

Karma's a bitch.

Back in the dressing room, I pulled on my jeans, T-shirt, and sweater, relieved at how, with each additional layer, I felt more and more like myself. I tossed the balled-up hospital gown into the hamper. At the check-out desk, a nurse handed me a small baggie of ice for the pain and swelling.

Outside, the sky was dark and the temperature hovered near freezing. I didn't know it yet, but this was the first of many days that would be lost to cancer, a disease that siphons time, energy, and life. I settled in the passenger seat and slipped the cold pack into my bra. Later that night, unable to sleep, I would slip out of bed and into my office where, bathed in the white glow of technology, the Internet told me that, as a woman in her thirties with no family history of the disease, my risk of being diagnosed with breast cancer was 1 in 233. I turned off the light and tiptoed back to bed where, lying next to Mary, I nudged the odds even lower by taking into account the twenty years I'd been a strict vegetarian and the ten-plus years of yoga and meditation.

Surely that counted for something, right?

CHAPTER 3

The next day I had a phone interview with Dr. Christiane Northrup, one of my favorite celebrity docs. She'd written several *New York Times* bestsellers about women's sexuality. She was brilliant and insightful, outspoken and articulate. She had a rapid-fire brain and a wit to match. Interviewing her felt like chasing an avalanche downhill—the more she talked, the faster she spoke, with me racing to keep up. Because she was clear, quirky, and confident, she was infinitely quotable—a magazine writer's dream.

I was fourteen years old when I found a dog-eared copy of *Seventeen* magazine beside my older sister, Ginny's, four-poster bed. In the slick, glossy pages, with the smudge of black ink on my fingertips, the cotton-candy whiff of perfume ads, and the whispered intonations of female friendship, I fell in love. Imagining my byline appearing in their pages, I began to write. High School English and journalism teachers encouraged me, and my college decision was based solely on its journalism school. My degree from the University of Missouri, Columbia, was in magazine journalism, which led to internships, a staff position, and finally enough contacts to freelance. By age thirty, I had the only job I'd ever wanted—writing for women's magazines.

My job was my superpower. Outside of work I was shy, content to be on the outskirts of conversations, reserving my questions for private mulling. But an assignment emboldened me to pick up the phone and interview endowed chairs of medical departments at top universities;

bigwigs at the FDA, CDC, and NIH; executive directors of national women's health organizations; and celebrity doctors. No one was too big or too powerful. Without hesitation, I called them all. Women had questions, and it was my job to get answers. I wasn't cocky. I was self-assured. Mine was a purposeful confidence that came from loving a job and doing it well.

That afternoon, working on a story for a popular lifestyle magazine, I asked Dr. Northrup about her latest book on women's sexual power—how to cultivate it when you're young and let it ripen as you age. As predicted, she riffed in her brilliant but zany way on everything from why women should watch more soft porn to the importance of mutual masturbation on a couple's quest for intimacy.

Under normal circumstances, I was a fast and accurate typist. My brain's executive function was nimble enough to talk with my source in real time, queue up the next three questions, and keep one eye on the clock, plus an eye on where the interview needed to land to give the piece closure. But today my fingers stumbled across the keys. Typos and half-finished sentences piled up on the screen. She gave me her talking points on the importance of intimacy, loving your body, and sexual satisfaction, but my follow-up questions refused to come. That damn lump had hijacked my brain.

What if it was cancer?

What would breast cancer do to my sense of intimacy with Mary?

What if I stopped feeling sexual?

What if Mary lost interest in me?

The beady red light on my digital recorder assured me the interview wouldn't be a total loss. Afterward, shaky and unnerved by the failure of my superpower, I strayed across the hall to share interview highlights with Mary. We'd had several talks about how it was not okay for me to park myself in her office without asking, but where was the fun in that? Mary was at her desk with her back to the door. Elbows tucking into her ribcage, fingertips pecking at keys. In three steps, I crossed the room. Her faux-leather chair sighed under my weight. "Christiane Northrup says we need to ditch our vibrator."

What was the matter with me?

Why didn't I tell her I was scared about breast cancer? About the lump ruining our sex life? No doubt, if I had voiced my fears, Mary would have swiveled in her chair, scooted toward me, taken my hand, and told me that—no matter what—she'd be attracted to me and that our love would survive.

Instead, I kept at it. "She told me vibrators are overstimulating. Did you know the clit has eight thousand nerve endings? Honey, we gotta cut back."

Truth. We'd both been busy and stressed, a libido-killer that led us to reach for a vibrator out of expedience. For the first few years of our relationship, we'd had slow, luxurious sex. But, as the years wore on, busy schedules got the better of us. On average, it takes twenty minutes for a woman to climax. Multiply that by two and, well, lady love is a time commitment. Who has that kind of free time?

Mary erupted in a dismissive snort. She was immune to such proclamations because she knew they were short-lived. For instance, every nutrition story I wrote became my obsession du jour. Meat, processed foods, and dairy were purged from our kitchen early. Sugar, white rice, and gluten followed. In ten more years, I'd start eating all those things again. But, back then, I still thought diet might protect me from things like cancer. The desire to control one's life by controlling one's eating habits was hard to shake.

Undeterred by her body language, I plunged ahead, "She said women need to practice feeling intense pleasure throughout the body, not just in erogenous zones."

"That's ridiculous," she chuckled.

"She says women need to learn how to get turned on with less and less stimulation. That people are too focused on breasts and genitals. Honey, we've got to branch out."

"Please close the door on your way out," Mary said, refusing to break her gaze away from her screen.

I slouched back to my office, closed the door, and swung around to face the task at hand—transcribing the interview. Bored by the thought, my eyes moved to the bookshelves lining the walls, the heavy white corner desk anchoring the room, the butter-yellow file cabinet filled with hundreds of file folders—years of articles written for dozens of magazines—and landed on my favorite distraction, the dog.

Emma sighed and rolled over as my short fingernails crisscrossed her clammy belly, stirring up dog hair and salty scent. Crouching next to her dog bed, my eyes caught on a magnet that had fallen off my filing cabinet, and a wave of nostalgia swept over me. The cheap black-and-white rectangle, the kind that looked like a business card, was from Osento, the women's bathhouse in San Francisco.

At age twenty-five, I moved to San Francisco for an internship at *Mother Jones*. One of my roommates told me about a women-owned, women-only bathhouse in the Mission, the city's Latino neighborhood. She scribbled the name on a piece of scrap paper, and I called information for the address—955 Valencia Street.

As a new arrival in 1990s San Francisco, I didn't know that Valencia Street was the corridor of queer grrl culture. I didn't know that, in another year, my annual salary as a full-time fact-checker at *Sunset Magazine* would be $34,000, enough to pay $625 a month for a studio apartment at Valencia and 18th Streets, the neighborhood's epicenter. That I'd savor the writing and performance art of Michelle Tea, who would publish a memoir about dyke culture in the city and call it *Valencia*. That I'd live a block from the city's last-standing lesbian bar, the Lex. I had no idea that Mary, a cute twenty-something grad student also lived in the Mission. It would be three more years before we'd meet.

My hunt for the bathhouse took me past auto-repair shops, appliance dealers, taquerias, sushi joints, and hair salons. Expecting to see a business facade, I passed the unremarkable gray Victorian twice before noticing the discrete house number. I climbed the stairs, pushed the doorbell, and waited with my stomach churning.

What the hell was I doing here?

A Catholic girl from Louisville, Kentucky, I had a polite, long-distance relationship with my body. It was down there, but we didn't talk much. Both of my parents had been private about their bodies. Even in her bedroom, my mother was never in anything less than a full slip. My father wore a camel-colored bathrobe on weekend mornings. A few times, I'd seen him in the thin cotton T-shirt and shorts he called "his BVDs."

On a balmy February evening in San Francisco, I didn't know what had drawn me to Osento other than wanting to know myself better and seek the community of women.

Was it too late to turn around?

The door swung open.

A compact person in a sweatshirt and faded Levi's motioned me inside. Later, I'd learn that her name was Sheila, and she was part watchdog, part den mother. She circled back behind a wooden teacher's desk. I stepped into a narrow entryway. On the floor were two dozen pairs of shoes. Frayed Converse, Doc Martens with hangdog tongues, Birkenstocks with crumbling cork. Each lined up side-by-side like so many obedient dogs.

"You here for a soak?"

I nodded.

Sheila handed me a clipboard with a sign-in sheet. Sinking onto a threadbare loveseat, I filled in my information and took a minute to look around. On my right was a bulletin board wallpapered in hand-written roommate-wanted signs, posters advertising Northern California music festivals, and local flyers for massage therapists, midwives, shamans, energy healers, and herbalists. Straight ahead was a curtain separating the foyer from the rooms beyond.

A peek through the fabric panels revealed a room with high ceilings and tall windows. The room was carpeted, the floor dotted with inflatable cushions where women lounged in various stages of dress and undress. Some napped, others meditated, a few spoke in hushed tones. Candles flickered in the fireplace. The air was scented with lavender, eucalyptus, and chlorine. The mood was neither prim nor lusty but instead felt relaxed and open.

"That'll be nine dollars, plus a buck for a locker. Cash only," said Shelia.

I pulled a wrinkled ten-dollar bill from my wallet, which she smoothed onto a stack of cash in a cigar box. Then she dropped the box into the open desk drawer, locked it up, and rose to her feet.

"Ready for the tour?"

Nodding, I slipped off my thrift-store combat boots and added them to the lineup. As we walked through the living room, my glance bounced between carpet and bodies. Svelte and taut, soft and jiggling, furry and waxed.

Sheila showed me a kitchenette in the far corner with filtered water, a bowl of fresh lemons, cutting boards, and knives for slicing. Then she led me to a swinging wooden door at the back of the living room and motioned me into a steam-filled room. Women lazed in and around a huge hot tub. Bodies bobbed, breasts floated, tattoos rippled beneath the water like tropical fish. On the tub's wide edge, women rested, piercings flashed, and steam rose from flushed bodies. Ceramic tiles covered every surface, including the walls and ceiling, from which drops of hot moisture would plunk down on bare skin.

Sheila pointed to the restroom and a door that led to a small meditation room before taking me into the house's backyard. The largest feature of the tiny patio was a wooden staircase. The stairs served a practical function—an emergency exit from the house's upstairs apartment—and a gathering place for bathers who ascended the steps to laze on a skinny deck. On the patio's ground level, tucked under the deck

29

and stairs, were two miniature wooden saunas: one wet and one dry. Miniature because each resembled an oak barrel turned on its side. To enter, you opened a small door and stepped into the barrel-shaped structure. Two facing bench seats fit four women comfortably and six women check-to-cheek.

Soon, this outdoor space would become my favorite retreat in the city. Inside the saunas, temperatures soared, water hissed on hot rocks, Epsom salts poured into outstretched palms, and bodies were sanded smooth. The moisture-thickened air filled with gossip. Who was sleeping with who. Who got fired from her job. Whose roommate was having a torrid affair. Between the stories, the darkness, and the dual sense of anonymity and community, my shy, wallflower self felt at home. Only when my body was near combustion did I push through the barrel's tiny wooden door, tiptoe across the patio, and ease into the icy cold-plunge. Near the end of every visit, I'd climb the wooden staircase and stretch out naked on the narrow deck. Cocooned in the warmth of my community, my eyes scanned the San Francisco sky for stars and my ears picked up the strains of music from Valencia's roaming Mariachi bands.

But that night, I tagged at Sheila's heels until the muffled sound of the doorbell filtered through the house and she excused herself. Retracing my steps to the living room, I stopped in front of the dented metal lockers. A part of me wanted to make an excuse about forgetting my loofa and leave. I didn't fit in. I wasn't cool enough to be here. I wasn't tattooed or pierced. I'd never hung out, in the nude, with strangers. But I wanted more for myself and my body than what I'd been taught to expect. So, on that first night, I shushed my nerves and I stayed.

Looking back on the night my twenty-six-year-old self entered Osento, I was standing on the threshold between who I'd been raised to be and who I wanted to become: a person who was free in her body. In the six years I frequented the bathhouse, its clientele—both straight and queer—taught me by example how to embrace my small breasts, my thick middle, my stocky legs, and my Scotch-Irish nose. They modeled a sense of unapologetic comfort in their bodies regardless of color, shape, or size. The body confidence I gained wasn't pride or self-satisfaction but a sense of deep gratitude. A comfort and ease that came with knowing who I was in this body of mine.

CHAPTER 4

Two days after my mammogram, at four o'clock in the afternoon of January 28, 2009, snowflakes the size and shape of communion wafers fell on Bloomington. Sitting at my desk listening to the staccato tap of Mary's productivity, the phone rang. It was my friend Lucy, the owner of the yoga studio where I taught on Wednesday nights. She was calling to talk about whether we should cancel class.

My caller ID clicked. I pulled the phone away from my face and squinted at the screen. St. Vincent's. I told Lucy I'd have to call her back and answered.

"This is Jana from the mammography center. Is this Catherine Guthrie?"

My heart stopped.

"I'm calling with the results of your biopsy."

My eyes closed. Jana's tone was all-business. That didn't bode well.

I pressed the phone's sweaty, oil-slicked plastic against my right ear.

The tapping from Mary's office stopped. She'd known I was expecting the call and had heard the subtle shift in my voice. The tension that comes from bracing oneself. Click, clack, click, clack. The wheels of her office chair rolled across the hardwood floor. Then the loose floorboard in the hall creaked under her weight.

"Your core needle biopsy tested positive."

I held my breath.

Mary hovered in the doorway.

"I'm sorry, but it's cancer."

A weight landed on my chest, pushing me back against the chair.

Just like that, one word upended my world—my perception of myself, my body, and my future.

I looked over my shoulder at Mary. Her face crumpled. Jana's words pelted me through the pinholes in the receiver. I turned back to my desk in a hurry to catch them, secure them to the page before they were lost in the blur of the moment. Words like cancer, positive, and surgeon. Words I'd written hundreds of times in articles about sickness, about disease, about other people, but never in reference to myself. Tears blurred my vision, making the black ink look smudged on the page.

My first thought was the most obvious: How can this be happening?

I'd done everything right. I fashioned an entire journalism career around learning how to avoid cancer, as if knowledge would spare me. Thanks to magical thinking, I was convinced I would sidestep chronic illness, as if disease was a blind alleyway healthy people willingly turned down.

Jana had already faxed the biopsy results to my doctor. She told me to call Dr. F's office to follow up. I nodded into the receiver.

In the corner, Emma slept, none the wiser. Outside the snow kept falling. Everything was as it was before, but everything looked different.

How was this conversation supposed to end? What are you supposed to say to the person who has just told you that you have cancer?

"Thank you?" I said.

I stood up and Mary pulled me close.

Have I mentioned that Mary stands an inch taller than me? That her shoulders are broad, like a swimmer's? That she has a half-dozen tattoos marking milestones in her life? That she is badass? That when she wraps her arms around me, I feel tucked in, like a card snug in its envelope?

"Should I call Lucy and let her know you can't teach tonight?"

I nodded. It was too early for words.

My feet took me down the hall and into our bedroom. I slid into bed and curled into a ball. A few minutes later Mary joined me, wrapping her arms around me. Outside, dropping temperatures and climbing winds transformed the snow from floating wafers into dive-bombing ice pellets. Later, the *Herald-Times* would report it to be Bloomington's worst snowstorm in thirty-one years.

But the day wasn't over. Jana had told us to see Dr. F for more details. And so we got in the car and went.

Dr. F's waiting room, typically filled with feverish children and bleary-eyed adults, was empty. A handful of women looked up from behind the reception desk as we blew in on a wintery gust.

"We got a call from St. Vincent's," said Mary.

The women exchanged glances. One grabbed a manila folder from the desk already tabbed GUTHRIE, CATHERINE. "Yes, she's expecting you." Mild confusion erupted. This wasn't a routine visit. Did they need to get my weight? Blood pressure? Twenty-five-dollar co-pay? Dr. F appeared, and they scattered like clucking hens.

The doctor's white sleeve extended toward an empty exam room. The light flickered on. Mary and I shuffled inside and took up two chairs against the wall. The scent of bleach stung my sinuses. The place had clearly been cleaned and closed for the day. Maybe we should leave and come back tomorrow?

Too late. Dr. F grabbed a stool, rolled it so close our knees nearly kissed. Today her long brown hair looked impossibly girlish, her face too young, too kind to deliver bad news. No one went into family medicine to dole out cancer diagnoses.

She repeated the day's news: my biopsy tested positive for invasive ductal carcinoma, meaning the cancer had started in a milk duct, gnawed through it like rust through a pipe, and seeped into the breast tissue beyond. How far had the cancer crept? It was too early to say. Mary's hand squeezed mine, the way mine squeezed hers during scary movies. The doctor's words bounced off me like rubber-tipped darts. This diagnosis was not mine. Surely this news was meant for someone else. Someone who hadn't dedicated her career to telling women how to avoid this very fate.

"The good news is we caught it early. You'll most likely be able to take care of it with a lumpectomy and radiation. Do you have a surgeon in mind?"

WTF? We'd just heard the news. Did other people keep lists of cancer surgeons on hand just in case?

"A couple of local surgeons operate on breast cancer," she said, before lowering her voice to a conspiratorial level. "But, if I were you, I'd go to Indianapolis."

Fifty stark miles of state highway sat between Bloomington and Indianapolis. The travel alone would leach hours of time and energy. A low-voltage current of anger ran through me. Anger at our dinky town, anger at the lump.

Dr. F handed me two prescriptions—one for anxiety and one for insomnia—and we shared a round of awkward "good luck" hand-shakes. As Mary and I left the colorless office, I was already nostalgic for Dr. F and her earnest, small-town family practice. I didn't know what my future held, but I suspected my diagnosis would catapult me into the big league of medical care—a life of big city hospitals, special-ists, and complex medical protocols. And I was right.

But, for now, the cancer diagnosis was so disturbing that, upon hearing the news, I couldn't imagine spending another second tending to life's ordinary concerns. I had cancer. How could I possibly eat dinner? Brush? Floss? Immediate medical action felt warranted. But having cancer was not like having chest pains or uncontrolled bleeding. There was no emergency per se. Oh, but how I yearned for competent-looking people in white uniforms to burst into our house, put me on a stretcher, and speed me away in an ambulance with flashing lights and a siren. I wanted to be elsewhere until the emergency passed. Until all was right in the world—the heart's artery bypassed, the bleeding stopped. I didn't want to bring the emergency home where it would seep into the walls, the rugs, and the brown couch and unravel my sense of safety. But that was not to be the case. No matter how alarming, a diagnosis of cancer was a nonemergency. There are steps, protocols, tests, and scans. This new life would have two speeds: hair on fire and monotony.

I have a knack for health trivia. Occupational hazard, I suppose. Here are a few facts:

- Mine was the most common type of breast cancer—invasive ductal carcinoma (IDC for short).
- Before a person can feel a breast lump, it must be at least one-centimeter wide.
- One centimeter's worth of breast cancer equals one billion cancer cells.
- Doctors told me later that my lump had been growing for roughly ten years.
- In that time, my lump grew its own network of blood vessels to manage nourishment and waste.
- By the time my tumor was detected, it may have been shedding cancer cells into my blood and lymph for years, like millions of seeds aloft on a breeze.
- Cancer seedlings, called micrometastases, are tough to spot until, like dandelions, they are a foot tall and waving their sunny heads at you from across the yard.
- Once breast cancer has spread, it is incurable.
- "Metastatic breast cancer kills six thousand women under the age of forty-nine every year, more than the number of AIDS-related deaths at the height of the crisis and twice that of the annual deaths of polio at the height of that

crisis," according to the author of *Malignant: How Cancer Becomes Us*, Lochlann S. Jain.

As for the events of that first night, I don't remember what happened. Most likely we went to the drugstore. Filled the prescriptions. Ordered take-out for dinner. Was I hungry? Probably not.

My singular memory is of Mary building a fire. I loved the fireplace in our living room. The hot, dry heat. The wavy dance of orange and yellow light. Emma flopping down at the edge of the hearth, her soft ears flickering at the fire's occasional crackle and spit. But, earlier that week, either Mary or I must have closed the chimney's damper against the winter chill because what started as a small stream of white, vapory smoke roiling out from the fireplace's upper lip grew into plumes of soot-filled storm clouds hovering near the ceiling.

Mary grabbed the poker from the hearth and stabbed at the burning logs, ransacking the pyramid she'd so carefully constructed. I leapt off the brown couch and threw open the room's many windows and doors in hopes of preventing what came next . . . the wail of the smoke detector.

Somewhere in the chaos of the shrieking alarm, the snowflakes gusting through the front door, Emma barking, and Mary swashbuckling with the fireplace, I lost my shit. I had cancer. I was breathing smoke. The house was full of fumes. There was no escape. I saw in the smoke every carcinogen, seen and unseen, that had snuck into my body over the years.

How could I have been so careless?

How could I have let this happen?

I shoved my mouth into the crook of my arm, took shallow sips of air, and cried.

During the next two years, the broad strokes of that evening would play out again and again. Me swept up in the invisible threat and unpredictable terror of breast cancer and Mary thinking she could fix it if she just tried hard enough.

CHAPTER 5

"Can-cer," Mary enunciated into the phone. "Catherine. Has. CAN-CER."

Three days after the diagnosis, we were barreling down I-65 at eighty miles per hour on our way to Louisville.

The largest city in Kentucky, Louisville sat on the banks of the Ohio River, a meandering waterway separating southern Indiana from Kentucky. My siblings and I had been raised to poke fun at our neighbors to the north. Hoosier jokes and insults, along the predictable lines of "Hoosier mamma?" taunts, were common at St. Leonard, my Catholic grade school. My parents underscored the lesson by pointing out Indiana plates on cars that were going too fast, too slow, or making an illegal U-turn. "See, it's those darn Hoosiers," my father would say, firming his grip on the wheel of the Lincoln Town Car, his four children lined up in the back seat like birds on a wire. It wasn't until I left home that I found out Kentucky, not Indiana, was the butt of most hick jokes.

"Catherine has cancer!" Mary repeated.

Fighting the urge to shoot her an "are you kidding me right now?" look, I stared straight ahead and reminded myself that Mary was doing her best to right my crooked world. My parents were leaving for Florida the next day. They'd be gone for six weeks, an annual migration they'd adopted upon retirement. To them, it was just another winter trip. In breast cancer parlance, six weeks felt like an eternity. Everything or nothing could happen in the next six weeks.

When Mary heard me say I wanted to see my folks before they left town, she'd jumped into action and planned a weekend trip. She'd made dog-sitting arrangements and even found someone to clean our house while we were gone—a surprise for me upon our return. And who could blame her for phoning a friend who lived in Louisville? She'd asked her friend if they could meet up for coffee the next day. Now, Mary was trying to explain to her the reason for our unplanned visit, and the weak cell service in Columbus, Indiana, was making a mess of the connection. Her friend caught every third word, but I heard Mary loud and clear. Her voice streaked with low-grade desperation. No doubt she needed the company of an old friend as much as I needed the familiar sight of my parents, but couldn't she find another way to phrase things?

It's hard to imagine a person who hasn't packed the word "cancer" with visceral scraps of pain, suffering, fear, and loss. And now the word was forever attached to me, branded on my body, and Mary couldn't see that the wound was still fresh.

The drive between Bloomington and Louisville was done on muscle memory. Seventy odd miles to the south—past Seymour, Vienna, and Blue Lick, farms gave way to urbanity. First came single-story strip malls, then two-story motels. Then crest a short ridge and a handful of skyscrapers materialize on the horizon. Louisville's middling skyline never looked better to me than when we lived in small-town Indiana. From downtown, hook a right, go three miles, exit at Grinstead Drive, take a quick left, rattle up a brick hill, and that's where my parents lived.

They'd been in the same house for thirty years, a one-hundred-year-old Victorian on Peterson Avenue in Crescent Hill. One of Louisville's oldest neighborhoods, Crescent Hill was a place where octogenarian oaks canopied the streets, red-brick cobblestone peeked through thinning asphalt, and front porches were built wide enough to double as front parlors during humid summers. My parents' house had all those things plus three stories, five fireplaces, and a sweeping staircase that figured prominently in our family's weddings and Christmas photos. My siblings and I called the house the Peterson Palace and only half in jest.

My parents had bought the yellow-brick house in 1980 as a fixer-upper when I was ten. The once proud home had been spliced into several apartments and occupied by a rotating cast of students from the nearby Southern Baptist Seminary. Hoping to restore it to its original grandeur, my father pulled out his checkbook and my mother rolled up her sleeves. Every weekday, he'd march down the stairs in a crisp, button-down she'd ironed the night before, his suit jacket hooked on a finger and slung over his shoulder. He'd head downtown and she'd pack us off to school and then spend the next six hours ripping out carpet, scraping off wallpaper, and stripping layers of paint from wood trim. At 2 p.m., she'd clean her tools, change her clothes, and start her second shift as kid chauffeur.

My mother valued hard work and stick-to-it-ness, traits she modeled as she transformed the old, segmented, neglected house into a unified home. She had little patience for the emotional neediness of children, and yet, we found ways to connect to her. Over time, living inside that house made me feel close to her, as if I'd managed to crawl back inside her skin, and no matter how far away my siblings and I moved, the house connected us to her in ways words never did.

But that dreary January day, it was my Uncle Bubba, not my mother, who met me at the back door. My mother's brother, Bubba was the uncle who picked his nose with the tab of a beer can just to get us kids laughing. The uncle who came to Thanksgiving dinner with a trick fork that, after everyone was served, he'd slyly telescope across the formal dining room table and spear a juicy slice of turkey off my mother's plate.

Now he had a long gray beard with a handlebar mustache. His beer belly was set off by red suspenders clamped onto sagging Levi's. A Marlboro dangled from his lips.

"How ya doin' kid!"

His grin smacked into me like a bird into a glass window.

"Kinda shitty. How 'bout you?"

I glared at the cigarette.

What part of carcinogens did he not understand?

He swept it out of his mouth and behind his back and bowed as I stepped through the door. The wooden screen door slapped shut as he went outside to help Mary unload the car. Three more steps put me at the threshold of the kitchen. My mother's hideout, bunker, and mission control. The kitchen's brick walls were two feet thick, which kept the room cool and gave it a Fort Knox–like sense of solidity and security. Three large windows let in the midday sun. Each deep plank of a window sill held collected treasures: cookbooks, faded greeting cards, a collection of bud vases with dainty cut flowers or sprigs of greenery. At the center of the room was an oval table and six chairs, six being the number of people in my family—my older sister, me, my brother, my younger sister, and my parents.

My mother loved to bake, and the two ovens were always exhaling sweet breaths of cookies, banana bars, and zucchini bread. She sipped a cup of hot Lipton all day and kept a teakettle on low heat on the range's front burner, the water popping and zapping against the kettle's insides like a live wire. In the winter, she used the oven the way other people used space heaters. She'd open the creaky door, turn the dial to bake at 350, pull up a chair, and read the *Courier Journal*. But today the kettle and the ovens were cold.

As I entered the room, my mother eased out from behind the table and gave me a series of gentle pats on the back. Oh how I wished we'd laid the groundwork for how to talk about pain. But we had no shared language, so we made do. I swallowed hard and brushed away a stray tear. "Think I'll go upstairs and lie down."

Mary bustled through the back door, a bag slung over each shoulder. She glanced up at me, her eyes anxious and quizzical.

41

"Stay and visit. I'm going upstairs to lie down a bit." I repeated.

The only good thing about a cancer diagnosis was that no one questioned your desire for a nap.

Climbing the narrow back staircase, I heard the scraping of chair legs on the wooden floor and the soft bump of the pantry door opening. Mary, my mother, and Uncle Bubba settling around the table for a snack of Wheat Thins and pimento cheese.

To get to my old bedroom on the third floor, take a sharp right at the top of the first flight of stairs and go through a narrow hallway of switchbacks to yet another staircase. On the long wall, my family's faces peered from photos hung salon-style. The black-and-white portrait of my parents as bride and groom. The sun-washed photo of Beth at six months old, all dimples and grin in a white-and-yellow Easter dress. And the last family portrait taken before my siblings and I scattered off to college.

In it, we all crowd around a yellow couch against a chalkboard-green backdrop. I'm wearing a sleeveless silk blouse and a long pencil skirt with a slit at the calf. My shoulder-length hair, the hair my parents always called "dishwater blonde" lest I feel special in a family of brunettes, shimmered with streaks of gold, because summer had just ended. I was seventeen. Posed on the arm of the couch, my hand on my mother's shoulder, my eyes gazing straight at the camera, I looked as if I knew how to inhabit a woman's body. What the photo didn't capture was the growing disconnect I felt between the person I was expected to be—a young woman who craved the attention of boys, who wanted to get married and have children—and the person taking shape on the inside. A person who'd rather stay home and read than go to a house party or a high school football game. Who wanted a life of adventure and freedom. A person who, when she kissed boys, felt nothing but obligation.

The following Monday, back in Bloomington, the bleat of the alarm clock rattled us out of bed before dawn. We groped for switches on bedside lamps and lay blinking at the ceiling. Night pressed against the windows. What was so urgent that it required us rising before dawn? Oh, right, Catherine has cancer.

The world was upside down. Last week I'd been a magazine journalist, someone paid to write about breast cancer with professional distance and objectivity. Now I'd been pushed out of the press box and onto the playing field.

The week before, we'd thrown ourselves into the task of surgeon shopping with the zeal of two people eager for distraction. Mary had reached out to her friends and colleagues, and it wasn't long before the name of a female breast cancer surgeon with an excellent reputation surfaced.

When I'd called, the scheduler's voice had been businesslike, confident, reassuring. Could we be there at 7 a.m. Monday morning? Of course, what else did we have to do? Cancer trumped all—Mary's class prep, my deadlines, our life together. What couldn't wait for cancer? Last week's urgencies were this week's follies. I'd gotten off the phone with a sense of calm and clarity.

But now, in the deep-space dark of an early-February morning, everything felt jarring. The teakettle whistled. The toaster popped. The water in the bathroom surged from the faucet as teeth were brushed and faces washed. The shotgun sound of the storm door was followed by the revving of the car. Our ruckus threatened to wake the neighborhood from its deep winter sleep.

Inside the car, Mary's pale cheeks flamed red from the cold, her glasses steamed, a fringe of hair stuck out, like a tongue. She wore her blue wool cap, the one with the earflaps that end in braids and make her look like a butch Pippi Longstocking.

On the road, white noise filled the car—a blend of tire hum, heater breath, and low-toned news anchors on NPR. The scent of stale dog drifted from the backseat even though we'd left Emma at home. In the coming months, when the weather cooperated, we'd bring her along. She loved her "crate on wheels," and her wiggles and soft cries of joy whenever we returned to the car were a welcome counterweight to the seriousness of tests and treatments. Her presence also gave us a practical reason to punctuate the end of every doctor's visit with a walk in a nearby park or even a strip of grass at the edge of the parking lot. But this morning was too early and too cold for dogs.

My feet slipped out of my blood-red Dansko clogs and tucked under me into a cross-legged seat. My winter coat stretched taut over my knees like a down bubble. Mary and I rode in silence, each lost in the storm cloud of her own concerns.

Shopping for a breast cancer surgeon felt like a high-stakes version of the Mystery Date board game I played with my sisters growing up. Would the surgeon and I mesh? Was she someone with whom I could envision a lasting relationship? Could I imagine her slicing into me?

When I thought about meeting the surgeon, I got the same fluttering in my stomach as when my eight-year-old self leaned over the game board, reached for the white plastic door, and pinched its tiny doorknob—no bigger than a thumbtack. Behind the door was my mystery date. My jaw clenched to deflect my sisters' giggles should I draw the Dud.

The surgeon's office was forty-five minutes away, in Greenwood, Indiana, a suburb on the south side of Indianapolis. Dr. L was the only woman I would interview for the job. As cliché as it sounds, I'd hoped a female surgeon might be more empathetic. That she and I would click by the sheer coincidence of our shared gender. But as soon as Mary and I entered Dr. L's office, my confidence flagged. I don't remember what I noticed first—was it the pink carpet, the pink curtains, or the pink upholstery? Or maybe the pink lab coats worn by the staff, each name badge festooned with tiny pink ribbons?

My vision hazed. The high-pitched buzz of the fluorescent lights became a hive of angry bees swarming behind my eyes. This was a mistake. I wanted to grab Mary's hand and pull her out the door, into the parking lot, back to the safety of the car. But she'd taken a seat and pulled out a book. She didn't seem to be having the same misgivings.

What was my problem?

I swam across the sea of pink carpet, picked up the pen, and added my name to the patient roster. As I joined Mary in the pink chairs, a sense of dread spread across my chest, as if I'd pledged a sorority I had no desire to join.

In hindsight, I should have been prepared for the pink. I knew about pink ribbons and Pinktober. I knew the color of little girls had been co-opted to sugarcoat the disease that killed their mothers, grandmothers, and aunts. I'd read and cheered "Welcome to Cancerland," Barbara Ehrenreich's seminal critique of the "relentless bright-siding" of breast cancer published in *Harper's Magazine* in 2001. But, until that moment, the privilege of good health had allowed me to look the other way. As a woman's health journalist, I had plenty of battles to choose from—let someone else deal with the pink ribbon bullshit.

Again with the karma.

A nurse led us to an exam room where a woman in her early sixties with frosted hair and pancake makeup stood with her hands clasped in front of her waist. The nurse introduced her as Sharon, my nurse navigator. Sharon was a breast cancer survivor who would sit in on my appointments, said the nurse. Sharon would talk with me about my options and make sure I didn't get confused.

Hot pinpricks of defensiveness rose up my spine. My eyes narrowed at what I interpreted as condescension.

Are testicular cancer patients assigned male survivors to sit with them and hold their hands? My sexist-bullshit meter was ringing off the hook.

Sharon's eyes, thick with black liner, met mine. "Welcome to the sisterhood."

My nostrils flared.

Her lips stretched across her face like a thin pink balloon in the moment before a clown inflates it, twists it into the shape of a poodle. I wanted to slug her.

Mary made the first move. "Thanks, I've got this," she said to Sharon as she corralled her toward the open door.

"Are you sure?" said Sharon.

"Yup."

She held the door open with one hand and eased Sharon out with the other. The rat-a-tat of my pulse slowed.

My cancer diagnosis had dredged up some ugly insecurities. I'd raced to judge Sharon before she could judge me. In Sharon's stick-straight spine, painted-on smile, and pink-ribbon bejeweled outfit I saw an enforcer of the feminine code, rules I'd bucked all my life. Women were supposed to smile, wear makeup, shave their legs, be passive, marry men, and bear children. I labeled her as someone who wouldn't under-stand me, my relationship with Mary, my tomboy-femme approach to womanhood. I could barely outrun the enforcers of heteronormativity when I was healthy. How could I evade them when I was sick?

With the door closed, I could start undressing. Sharon had laid out a gown for me on the exam table. Thinking about how we'd rushed her out the door made me feel like an asshole.

Sharon had been doing her job. She was just there to help. Why couldn't I just accept help where help was offered?

Mary heard my thoughts. "Honey, Sharon will get over it," she said folding my sweater and T-shirt into a neat pile. "You're the patient. This is your show. You get to decide who stays and who goes."

Oh, how I wanted to believe her!

A few minutes later, Dr. L swept into the room. She looked to be in her fifties. Her straw-colored hair was pulled into a tidy ponytail. She had a caffeinated energy and a clipped manner. A few pleasantries were exchanged before she shoved my mammogram from St. Vincent's onto the wall-mounted light board and scrutinized the bruise-colored film.

With a yank and a clang she pulled out the exam table's metal extension. I swiveled my legs up and lay back. She folded the thin cotton gown to reveal my left breast. Her fingers began their circular dance.

I stared at the ceiling and pretended there was no place I'd rather be than on a padded table in a pink shrine in suburban Indianapolis at sunrise with a breast surgeon tunneling her fingers deep into my left armpit on a truffle hunt for swollen lymph nodes. How quickly cancer had stripped me of false modesty. The shift was underway—the shift of no longer thinking of my body as mine, as something private. My body was morphing into something that belonged to medical professionals, to people who "knew better."

Dr. L finished her exam and sank onto a padded stool with wheels that clicked softly as she rolled toward me. The black-and-white image of my left breast hovered over her right shoulder like a misshapen moon. She tore a sheet of paper from a pad on her lap, took a Sharpie from her pocket, and, in the empty white rectangle, drew a circle for my breast, a dot for the lump, and a straight black line for the incision.

Her words bounced off me like hail off a metal roof. Behind my eyes, my brain was reversing away from the conversation as if from an accident scene.

Clearly, I should have asked Sharon to stick around.

Thankfully Mary was capturing every detail as efficiently as my digital tape recorder.

"You'll need to find a plastic surgeon to finish the job," said the surgeon.

Wait. What plastic surgeon? Why did I need a plastic surgeon?

A lumpectomy sounded no more complicated than an appendectomy or a tonsillectomy—bits of unhealthy tissue removed and discarded. I'd had pre-cancerous moles removed, right? Was this really that different? My lump was no bigger than a rosary bead. Surely a plastic surgeon was overkill.

"You do have an oncologist, right?" quizzed the surgeon. "What about a radiation oncologist?"

Mary calmly flipped to a fresh page in her palm-sized notebook and jotted down the growing list of doctors we needed to shop for as dutifully as she would make a grocery list for tonight's dinner.

"Um," I stammered. "Radiation . . . so, is that really necessary?" A knot of panic wedged itself in my stomach.

"Yes, but don't worry, radiation tightens the skin around your breast," she replied. "It's like getting a breast lift."

This was the first of many times doctors would let me know how breast cancer treatment could improve my appearance.

I looked at my chest. My breasts were perky, peach-sized, barely a B cup. They were perfectly proportioned to my body. The skin was smooth, unmarred by scars or stretch marks. These breasts had never ridden the hormonal swells of pregnancy or faced the rigors of breast-feeding. Truthfully, they'd hardly known vigorous exercise. I may have been thirty-eight but my breasts didn't look a day over eighteen.

"Well, think it over." And with that Dr. L gave us a darting handshake and departed for her next patient. Mary and I looked at each other. We had a lot to figure out.

A few minutes later we were almost to the exit when a nurse came running up from behind us.

"You almost forgot your bag," she said, extending a white canvas tote with a pink trim.

"Oh no, that's not mine."

"It's a gift. Just a little something we like to send home with our new patients."

Having never gotten a parting gift from a doctor, I was suspicious, but I was raised to be polite. I knew I was supposed to take the bag and say "thank you"—so I did. A few minutes later as Mary steered back toward the highway, I opened the bag and pulled the contents into my lap: a pink pen, a pink water bottle, a pink day planner, and a pink journal.

Breast cancer swag? What was I supposed to do with all this shit?

I glanced sidelong at Mary. She shook her head at the Pepto-Bismol pile. We soon learned that breast cancer equaled tchotchkes. Pink knickknacks would rain down on me for the next two years. From that day onward, the color pink stuck to me like warm bubblegum on the bottom of a shoe.

Back in Bloomington, even with the pink freebies stuffed into a cardboard box in the hall closet, signs of cancer patient-hood crept into our home as stubbornly as the poison ivy that snaked through my flower beds. The number for St. Vincent's glared at me from the pad of paper by the phone. Young Survival Coalition brochures fanned across the dining room table. A three-ring binder stuffed with breast cancer basics and local resources courtesy of Bloomington Hospital squatted on the sideboard. My new best friends—Ativan and Ambien—sat on the shelf over the toaster. Seeing signs of cancer spread across the landscape of my familiar reminded me of another time I'd witnessed cancer's crawl into an otherwise vibrant-looking life.

Years ago, Mary and I drove to Atlanta to visit her half-sister Susan who was sick with ovarian cancer. We knew it was serious, but we didn't know it was end-stage. (Did we even know what "end stage" meant?) We didn't know she'd be dead within the month. Susan's two college-aged daughters invited us to spend the night with them in their mother's house. I'd never met Susan, but I liked her from the moment I walked through her door.

The energy of the house hummed with the vibration of a life well lived. Photographs of friends and family smiled at us from walls and tabletops. Cozy furniture invited us to curl up for conversation. French doors led to a brick patio where cardinals and chickadees gathered at bird feeders.

The four of us had settled into the living room to talk, when I noticed something else about the house. Scattered about the coffee table were a box of tissues, a sleeve of saltines, and a copy of *Chicken Soup for the Cancer Survivor's Soul.* Piled on a side table were unread magazines. A heating pad lay on the floor next to a recliner, the pad's cord curled to one side like a sleeping dog. I'd stepped over the threshold between the world of the healthy and the world of the sick. The private bubble of the chronically ill.

The steady march of cancer into a life may start with an innocent-looking pill bottle or a doctor's bill—as easy to overlook as the first vague symptoms. Then a stream of drug store supplies and piles of paperwork as illness takes root. And, in Susan's case, the final health crisis that transplanted her from home to hospital. I picture her preparing to leave, unplugging the heating pad and glancing out the window to see if her bird feeders were well stocked. How could she have known that she'd never come back?

And so it was I sat in my own house, surrounded by the first shoots of breast cancer's plantings. Where would it end? Would a naive young visitor sit on the brown couch a few months or years from today, her eyes widening as she cast her glance upon the medical detritus that swallowed me whole?

Darkness suffocated February's anemic sun by five o'clock. As the light waned, my worry-meter rose. Anxiety-prone by nature, cancer shot my angst into a new stratosphere. Ativan became my new bestie. The tiny white discs disintegrated on my tongue like the Smarties eaten by the dozens on Halloween nights of my childhood. But instead of sugar leaching into my bloodstream, it was Lorazepam, drugs that wrapped my nerve endings in thick, padded blankets. As long as Lorazepam was on board, nothing jarred, nothing jangled. Six years from that day, I would struggle to wean myself from Ativan's grasp, but I didn't know this yet, and the drug felt like magic.

On most nights Mary made a point of coming home by seven instead of the usual nine or ten. We'd hit the couch and zone out to whatever Netflix DVD had arrived in the mail that day. A friend had suggested we watch *Crazy Sexy Cancer*, a documentary by Kris Carr about her cancer experience. The movie arrived on a Friday and we decided to give it a look.

The scent of fresh popcorn filled the house, the dog trotted toward the kitchen to vacuum the popped kernels that inevitably hit the floor. I slid the movie out of its red sleeve and into the DVD player. Mary handed me a metal mixing bowl full of fluffy kernels, and we settled into the brown couch. Soon I was nurturing an intense and irrational dislike of Kris Carr.

Carr had long blond tresses, emerald green eyes, and a coltish figure. She was sexy. She was hip. She lived in New York City and was an aspiring actress who'd been diagnosed with a rare form of cancer. She bee-bopped and chitchatted through her CT scans and doctors' appointments with her quirky tribe of fun-loving friends and family members. Yes, okay, a few frames showed her in tears, but she was setting such a high bar of cancer-glam. How would I ever reach it?

My body fidgeted under the blanket. First one foot stuck out, then the other. I peeled off my socks and unzipped my hoodie. Still my skin was hot and itchy. "You okay?" Mary asked, her voiced laced with annoyance.

"Yeah," I lied.

"Wanna stop watching?"

"No," I replied, unwilling to own my bad attitude.

We watched as Kris got in shape and swore off sugar, salt, and alcohol. We saw her at the grocery store filling her cart to overflowing with green, leafy vegetables. She went vegan and bought a mini-trampoline. She suggested that clean eating and bouncing keeps cancer at bay. She fell in love with her handsome cameraman, who proposed on camera. (Of course!) The documentary ended with Kris princess-stepping down a rose-petal-strewn aisle, in a wedding dress, its plunging neckline revealing the contours of her perfectly shaped breasts.

As the credits rolled, Mary gathered the empty bowls, whistled for the dog, and went to the kitchen, leaving me in a sweaty, itchy heap on the brown couch. A part of me knows it's a sin to cast stones at women with stage 4 cancer, especially when they are making bank from a shitty situation. Carr masterfully played the cards she was dealt. But it wasn't Carr exactly that irked me. It was her inference that "clean living" could obliterate cancer. The one sure thing we know about cancer is that it's a complex, multifaceted monster of a disease. And most of us won't be saved by green smoothies.

CHAPTER 6

My next mystery date was with a general surgeon in Bloomington. His office was only a few short blocks away but still we drove. Sidewalks were coated with ice from last week's storm and a bone-chilling wind was kicking up.

Dr. H came recommended by my neighbor Lorraine. She and her husband Bob were close to my parents' age and lived across the street. Five years ago, the day after Mary and I moved in, they'd been the first to welcome us to the neighborhood and the first locals to challenge my stereotype about small towns and homophobia.

That day, I was unpacking clothes in the bedroom when I saw Bob and Lorraine sauntering toward our door. Him in a white polo and khakis, his gray hair neatly trimmed, a scrappy daisy bouquet in his hand. Her in a daffodil-yellow summer dress, carrying a bag of Beggin' Strips for the dog. They looked as if they'd come straight from church. I bit my lip and dropped the clothes on the bed.

"Um, hon?"

Mary didn't appreciate my paranoia about small towns, so I'd kept my worries to myself, but she needed to know we were about to come face-to-face with our first set of neighbors.

"Yeah?" she popped her head in the door. She had on her weekend uniform of a faded ball cap, an old college T-shirt, and L.L.Bean cargo shorts. I had on Levi's and Birkenstocks. We were two characters from Alison Bechdel's *Dykes to Watch Out For.*

Ding dong! BAARK BARRK BARKKKK—Emma beat us to the welcome.

Mary opened the door to a smiling Bob and Lorraine. They handed us the flowers and dog treats. We gushed thanks. Emma barked and sniffed Bob's crotch. We invited them into the living room, and for the next thirty minutes, we chatted amiably among the piles of cardboard and clouds of bubble wrap. Lorraine had an extroverted cheerfulness, a way of tossing her head back and chortling at the ceiling. Bob was quietly affable. They were Hoosiers born and bred. She managed a pet store, while he was a janitor.

Eager to prove myself as a good homeowner and a convivial neighbor, I told them about our plans to clean up the garden and rebuild the listing chimney. They told us about the best local dog runs, the neighborhood trash pick-up day, and how to get a city-issued blue recycling bin. On his way out the door, Bob lowered his voice and mentioned that his brother was gay, then gave us a toothy grin and a thumbs up in the way that older men sometimes do.

Bob and Lorraine couldn't have given a hoot about us being lesbians. They just hoped we'd be good neighbors—ones that picked up after their dog, took their trash to the curb and kept their recycling tidy. It was me who had rushed to judge them, eager to pigeonhole them as small-minded just because they lived in a small town.

In the following years, Lorraine and I settled into a routine of across-the-yard waves and mutual appreciation of one another's dogs. Hers yapped. Mine thundered. We had an unspoken dog-owners pact not to complain. Beyond dogs, I appreciated her "anything-is-possible-if-you-stick-to-your-guns" brand of Midwestern optimism, and she appreciated my green thumb.

The yard had become my escape when the pressure of Mary's work stress threatened to blow the roof off the house. That first summer, as Mary wrestled her doctoral dissertation into a book, I spent every hot, sticky afternoon pulling up Virginia creeper and poison ivy. Taking my mother's advice not to yank willy-nilly but to trace each vine deep into the ground before prying it off every rock, stump, and fence post, I dug deep so the roots would come out clean. Otherwise they would grow back even stronger, more invasive.

Gardening was a hidden doorway into my mother's inner world. When finished with the hands-on aspect of raising kids, she'd turned her focus and quiet energy to plants. She lovingly weeded, watered, and pruned her extensive garden at the Peterson Palace and, when she was done, tossed her tools in the car and drove to my older sister's house to weed her yard. Now, with a yard of my own, I was able to seek her input and advice, connecting over a shared project.

Twice a year, she drove up from Louisville with the back of her station wagon filled with a dozen or more grocery bags, each holding a green sprout and an accompanying rootball she'd unearthed that morning. Her castoffs were self-propagating plants—daylilies, hostas, and mums that had outgrown or overstayed their welcome in her yard. On the floor of her car's backseat would be a pitchfork with bent prongs and mud-caked tennis shoes. Together we pulled up vines, dug out stumps, edged flowerbeds, and planted pink peonies, purple cone flower, and rusty sedum. Along the side of the house, a dozen delicate, white candytufts outlined the edge of the stone wall, like a snow drift. The house was on a slight hill and the front yard had a three-foot-high rock wall that separated it from the sidewalk. Along the wall we planted armfuls of creeping phlox that bloomed a lavender waterfall every spring.

Working from home and gardening turned out to be a good match. When I needed a break, I'd walk out the front door and head straight for the weeds. Two minutes later my bare hands were filled with leaves, stems, and roots. So satisfying! When a nine-inch-long dandelion root slid up and out of the earth unbroken, a wave of accomplishment washed through me—a rush that was elusive with writing. The garden was also a bottomless receptacle for my anxiety. When worry threatened to unravel me, I'd head outside and yank, pull, and scratch at anything that didn't belong. As if, by ridding my flowerbeds of "other," I could oust it from myself. Was cancer other, or was it me?

As I made my way around the yard, I often saw Lorraine arrive home from work and head out to walk her two lap dogs. After a day of napping, the duo galloped down the sidewalk, straining at their halters, their little bodies bouncing with pure pleasure. Lorraine, in her color-coordinated track suit and thickly-cushioned cross-trainers, slow-jogged behind them, laughing and urging them on as if the concrete were tundra and Frankie and Carl her sled dogs in training. She'd disappear down the road but her whoops and hollers were carried back to me on the light summer breeze.

During those years of over-the-fence chitchat, Lorraine told me what it was like to ride shotgun to breast cancer. The disease had swept through four generations of her family, not unlike the late-summer tornadoes that sent all us Midwesterners running for our basements. Breast cancer had laid claim to her mother and her grandmother. And, more recently, her niece and three of her six sisters had been diagnosed and treated. Lorraine had a mammogram every six months and lived in a perpetual crouch waiting for the disease to take the first swing.

One early summer day, four years into our friendship, Lorraine sat stiffly in a lawn chair on her back patio. Her miniature Schnauzer, Frankie, was on her lap. As was my custom, I pulled a few weeds then wandered over to say hello. But Lorraine didn't look up or even turn her head. She told me she'd been at the doctor. Her latest mammogram showed a suspicious mass. As she spoke, her arms tightened around the gray-and-white dog. Frankie whined and licked her chin. Thumbs-up Bob had been gone a year. He'd left for a younger woman he'd met at church. I fumbled for words.

"I'm sure it's nothing."

Lorraine recoiled ever so slightly. My words had been as caustic as the salt I sprinkled on slugs that munched on my hostas. How I'd wanted to reel those words back in. But it was too late.

A week later, she told me the biopsy was positive. The mass was breast cancer. She'd marched into the local surgeon's office and asked for a double mastectomy without reconstruction. In the telling, her voice was resolute. "Good for you," I'd said.

After her surgery, she rang our doorbell. Reminiscent of the day she and Bob had stood in our living room and we'd all sized each other up as neighbors, she stood confident and strong. Her voice was filled with relief. "I'm so glad they're gone. Do you wanna see?"

My mind scrambled, not wanting to say the wrong thing. I looked at Mary. Her mouth was open in a half-smile, her eyebrows scrunched in confusion. Lorraine gathered her shirt from the bottom and raised it to her shoulders. Yep, this was really happening—she was showing us her naked torso. I winced. On her chest were two fresh scars. Hers was the first double mastectomy I'd seen in person.

Two years later, when I was diagnosed, I called Lorraine. She'd know what to do.

"Make an appointment with Dr. H," she said. "He'll do ya right."

I took her advice and made the appointment with the general surgeon.

At Dr. H's office, the walls were covered in dark wood paneling. A television the size of a washing machine crouched in the corner, and barrel-shaped club chairs lined the walls. Crawling across the moss-colored shag carpeting was a diaper-clad baby with a crusty nose. A man slept upright in a chair nearby, his dusty jeans and cap with a John Deere logo reminding me that, for many people in rural Indiana, Bloomington was the nearest big-city option for health care.

Twenty minutes later, Mary and I watched as Dr. H held my mammogram up to the light. So far, the surgeon-patient waltz mirrored the one I'd done that morning in Greenwood—with one difference. Before he started the physical exam, he called his nurse into the room. She stood silently in the corner, but her presence was palpable, like a security guard at a museum. I learned later that nurse chaperones are common when a male physician was doing a breast exam.

Dr. H did a perfunctory exam of my lump and nearby lymph nodes. Then he sat down, pulled out a piece of paper, and began to draw. Like the first surgeon, he illustrated how he'd cut out the lump. Again, I hoped to see something approximating a worm and an apple, but in his drawing, my post-lumpectomy breast looked more like a pizza with a slice missing.

"So, if this sounds okay, we'll go ahead and schedule the surgery for next week."

Whoa! Not so fast buddy.

I'd written a story for *Prevention* the year before about how to choose a well-qualified surgeon. I'd revisited my notes before that day's appointment and jotted down some questions. My experts had underscored the importance of avoiding general surgeons for complex cases. "Find a surgeon who specializes in the type of operation you need," they said. Dr. H was a general surgeon, not a breast surgeon, but I was considering him because Lorraine had spoken so highly of his work. Plus, his office was only two blocks from our house.

"I just have a few questions."

He looked at his watch.

Speaking up risked being labeled a "difficult patient," but I plowed ahead. "What percentage of your surgeries are breast-cancer related?"

His chair squeaked as it rolled away from me. He leaned back, crossed his arms, and narrowed his eyes.

"I operate on cancer all the time. Just did a lung cancer case yesterday, took out an entire lobe."

"Yes," I said, "but what about breast cancer?"

Not every general surgeon was well versed in breast cancer surgery. A lumpectomy wasn't just about removing the lump after all but also about checking the nearby lymph nodes. I worried that a mistake—either in removing the tumor or not taking out cancerous lymph nodes—could be fatal, not immediately but five, ten, fifteen years from now, when Dr. H would be happily ensconced in a retirement community in Phoenix. All solid cancerous tumors shed cells into blood and lymph, but breast cancer cells are notorious for hitchhiking to distant sites—the brain, lungs, and bones—and lying dormant for months, years, or even decades.

His back stiffened. "Bloomington is a small town, there aren't that many breast cancer patients."

"Yes, but how many, on average, do you do in a month?" I pressed.

Mary shifted forward in her chair, letting me know she had my back. I needed the support. My confidence was as thin as the paper gown I was wearing. Normally I had no problem asking doctors tough questions. I was a health journalist, for cripes' sake. But, from the seat of the patient, everything looked different.

"Maybe one or two," he sputtered. "I can't make a living off of breast cancer surgeries. I've got kids to put through college."

His eyes gleamed. He lowered his head and started writing something on my chart.

"Let's talk after your bone scan."

What? No one else had mentioned a bone scan, usually reserved for cases where doctors suspected the cancer had spread.

The sweat on my palms caused my hands to slip off the edge of the exam table.

"Your cancer may be stage 4 for all we know," he said. "I wouldn't want to operate until we're sure."

Mary slapped her notebook shut and shoved it into her backpack. "I think we're finished here," she said, handing me my shirt.

I don't remember the look on Dr. H's face as we hustled out into the cold sunshine. But I do remember that this man manipulated my fear to put me in my place, silence my questions, and cement his position of power. Unfortunately, it underscored my nagging distrust of surgeons.

When I was twelve years old, a routine physical was all that stood between me and two weeks of horseback riding camp in Midway, Kentucky. I'd been saving my babysitting money and dreaming of learning how to ride hunter jumpers, the camp's specialty. I was a healthy kid who played every sport my grade school offered—basketball, volleyball, track, and softball. This physical was going to be a breeze.

The last thing on the doctor's list was a scoliosis check. He asked me to touch my toes, then slid an authoritative finger down my spine. He stopped halfway. Clucked. Then started over at the base of my neck. My mother glanced up from the notes she was jotting on her grocery list. My doctor's appointment was just one of a dozen stops she would make that day.

"Looks like she's got a curve," he said.

Goose bumps sprang up on the backs of my arms. I'd learned about scoliosis from the Judy Blume book *Deenie*, about a girl my age who'd been diagnosed with a curvature of the spine. One scene in particular had given me nightmares for days—Deenie had to sit still while nurses wrapped strips of cold, wet plaster around her naked body. The plaster made a cast that Deenie had to wear everywhere—even to school! My twelve-year-old self had cringed with empathy and mortification. Now a doctor had used that word in reference to me. My hands shook as I laced my dirty white Keds. He gave my mom the name and number of a physical therapist. "Let's hope some back exercises will take care of it."

My tears didn't spill until my mom and I got to the parking lot. Standing on the oozing asphalt, the thin rubber soles of my tennis shoes turning to taffy, sniveling turned to a full-on bawl. My mother patted my shoulder and told me it would be okay. It wasn't.

I went to horseback riding camp. But at the end of the summer, X-rays showed the curve had gotten worse. The adults grew more concerned. As summer turned to fall, my mother added my twice-a-week physical therapy appointments to her giant desk calendar.

At the PT office, I'd lie on a scratchy brindle-colored carpet surrounded by exercise balls, rollers, and mats while a therapist showed me how to resist the pull of the curve. I did my exercises every night. Within weeks my back began to ache inconsolably. Sitting in the wooden desks at St. Leonard intensified the pain. I started popping Advil at recess, and by Halloween I'd moved on to prescription pain medication. By Thanksgiving I was lying on my parents' blue corduroy couch every afternoon, a heating pad pressed to my lower back.

My parents took me to an orthopedist. After taking more X-rays and asking lots of questions, he pronounced that a Milwaukee-style brace, the kind of back brace Deenie wore, was not an option because I'd finished my growth spurt. By the end of November, I had an appointment with a back surgeon. The surgeon ordered more X-rays. Even though my curve was mild and surgery wasn't indicated, he told my parents that the best way forward was a lumbar fusion. Two weeks later, I turned thirteen. My birthday gifts were geared toward a teenage shut-in: new pajamas, a Cabbage Patch doll, and a MASH calendar to mark the passage of time.

The surgery worked, and the surgery was a disaster. My parents drove me to the hospital just after Christmas of 1984. Both sat with me as presurgery checks and crosschecks were done. I learned to say "yes" if anyone in a white coat asked if I'd had a BM recently. I watched TV and played with the remote-control bed. Head up. Head down. Feet up. Feet down. After dinner, my father went home to put my siblings to bed. My mom would sleep on a cot next to my hospital bed. I was victorious at having scored some precious one-on-one time with my mother. It would be like a slumber party! But first we went for a slipper-shod walk after dinner when the activity of the hospital was winding down.

The corridor lights were dim. The air smelled of rubbing alcohol. The gummy rubber dots of the bottom of my hospital socks stuck to the linoleum. When we came to the two swinging doors marked "Intensive Care Unit," we hesitated. We'd been told that the ICU was where I would spend the first week of my two-week hospital stay. I shrugged. I was always up for an adventure. I liked new experiences, especially ones that got me out of school. I was too young to notice the nervous twitch behind my mother's eyes.

Memories of the days spent in the ICU are fuzzy. I couldn't talk or open my eyes, but my hearing was acute. As an eighth grader who'd read nearly every book in the grade school library, I aced most vocabulary tests, but that week I learned a raft of new words: chest tube, catheter, respirator, IV line, and morphine. Beside my bed, machines beeped, gurgled, and whooshed. As promised, a week after the surgery, I was transferred to the orthopedic surgery floor.

All other memories of my hospital stay are eclipsed by pain. My torso was heavy, dull, numb, shocked. My muscles sliced, a rib removed, a lung deflated, vertebrae rearranged. A scaffolding of metal rods and screws installed in my lumbar spine. To prevent bedsores, every thirty minutes, night and day, nurses came to roll me into a new position—left side, supine, right side. Each tug and pull spiraled me into new worlds of agony. I tried to be quiet. Crying out in pain slowed the process. The faster the nurse could fold, tuck, and position pillows the sooner the pain would lessen from a shriek to a dull roar.

Two weeks later paramedics carted me up the formal front staircase of the Peterson Palace on a stretcher. On the count of three they lifted me onto the bed, my body locked inside a clamshell brace. A legs-up turtle. The room would be my prison for the next three months, the brace for the next six. It wasn't the dreaded Milwaukee brace, but my brace did extend from my hips to my shoulders. It had a full back and breast plate that stabilized my spine while the bones knitted back together. For the next six months, I wore it twenty-four hours a day, except to shower. I hadn't escaped Deenie's fate after all.

After my fusion healed, my grandmother told me that if I wasn't careful, the rods would snap. She pursed her lips and shook her head. "It happened to my friend Martha. Broken rod poked right out of her back." Terrified, I spent my teenage years cowering on the sidelines of my life, watching as other kids ice-skated, roller-skated, and water-skied. Eventually, my lower back healed, the curve tamed. But we didn't know that correcting a lumbar curve can sometimes incite a new one in the middle or upper back. The body wants what it wants, and mine wanted to curve. By the time I was in my early twenties, a slight curve had formed between my shoulder blades, and my back began to ache.

In California, I got a job as a fact checker at *Sunset Magazine*. It was my first staff magazine job, meaning it came with full benefits, and I quickly made an appointment with a chiropractor in Menlo Park, a woman who was recommended by a coworker. I showed up to the appointment with X-rays of my hardware-filled spine. After hearing my health history and looking at the X-rays, she said the fusion had been totally unnecessary. She said my original back pain was most likely a muscle spasm caused by the exercises. "Back surgery was a fad in the eighties," she sighed, tapping her mechanical pencil on my X-rays. "Orthopedists fused everyone who came through the door." Since that moment, several other doctors have confirmed her assessment that my back surgery was overkill (at best) and dangerous (at worst).

That moment forever changed my view of surgeons—as flawed human beings, like the rest of us, who are taught to see patients through the prism of their schooling. Surgeries trend, just like fashion and music. And, like any other business, a surgical practice needs new customers.

Billboards on the highway near my parent's house in Louisville still heavily advertise the spine center and its surgeons, just as they did when I was a teenager. My parents had seen their child suffering, and I understand why they put me in the hands of a surgeon. What is harder for me to reconcile is how the surgeon neglected to prepare my parents (much less me) for the pain and immobility. Picture a thirteen-year-old girl lying flat in bed, open sores weeping from holes rubbed in her flesh by the metal brace, unable to sit or stand for three months. My mother's hushed voice on the phone in the next room reaches me, "I just had no idea. Why didn't they tell me how much pain she would be in? If I had only known . . ." In my mind, this is how the sentence ends, ". . . I would never have allowed this to happen."

No doubt, my becoming a health writer was fueled in part by wanting to help people understand the implications of their medical decisions. I wasn't anti-surgery. I had a much-needed tonsillectomy at age twenty-eight with a surgeon I trusted. But I was a wary consumer. I knew surgeons and patients often measured success differently. To the surgeon who operated on my spine, my case was a resounding success because I hit my recovery markers. But no one follows surgery patients long-term. This is a problem. What's more is that, as an adult, I knew the difference between hearing a surgeon describe an operation and the felt experience of living with the consequences. I had learned the hard way that just because surgeons can operate does not always mean that they should.

Now I was facing breast cancer surgery, and I wanted to get all the facts, make my own decisions, and above all choose someone I could trust. And that's why it is so hard to explain what came next.

On the evening of the dispiriting meeting with Dr. H, Mary and I were on the brown couch watching television when the phone rang. It was a friend who had a connection to one of the doctors who'd treated Lance Armstrong, the most famous cancer patient in America.

Wait? Was this a game cancer patients played: six degrees of separation from Lance Armstrong?

"No, really," she said. She told me that Lance's doctor practiced at Indiana University Medical Center in Indianapolis. She was school friends with his daughter. They'd just spoken, and the daughter had passed along her father's private email, inviting us to reach out to him to recommend a breast cancer surgeon.

I hung up and shot Mary a skeptical look.

"Why not just send him an email?" she said. "You've got nothing to lose."

And so I trudged upstairs, plunked down at my desktop, and typed an email to Lance Armstrong's cancer doctor introducing myself and my question: Who do you recommend for breast cancer surgery?

An hour later the phone rang again.

Holy shit, it was Lance friggin' Armstrong's doctor!

I clung to the receiver and got straight to the point. If he were in my shoes, who would he want to do the operation?

He didn't hesitate. "Dr. B."

The name was one I recognized. Dr. B was the director of breast surgical oncology at Indiana University Hospital. His name had come up when we googled breast cancer surgeons in Indianapolis. But we'd heard that access to him was limited. Rumors were that it took weeks to get an appointment. To avoid being disappointed, I hadn't tried. Lance Armstrong's doctor told me he'd make some calls and, in the meantime, to "feel free to drop my name as often as you need to." I thanked him and hung up feeling as if he had offered me a seat on the last lifeboat departing the Titanic.

At nine o'clock the next morning, I called Dr. B's office. In response to my question about scheduling a new-patient appointment, the voice on the other end replied with a polite "no can do." Then I dropped the famous doctor's name. Like a skeleton key, it opened all doors. Within ninety minutes of picking up the phone, I had an appointment.

Twenty-four hours later we were zipping along State Highway 37 on our way to see Dr. B. Beyond the car's windows, fields stretched in all directions, horizontal lines broken by the occasional clapboard farm house or dilapidated outbuilding. Every twenty minutes the highway slowed to a crawl through a one-stoplight town complete with a red brick high school, a car dealership, and a gun shop.

From the passenger seat, I stole a glance at the gas gauge, relieved to see it was half full. I loathed unplanned stops, especially at isolated gas stations. I considered standing outside the car on a slab of concrete in the middle of nowhere, an invitation for a hate crime. Was my paranoia because I was a woman? A lesbian? A lesbian traveling with her partner?

I'd never been physically hurt, but I'd been on the receiving end of countless verbal assaults. The word *dyke* was a perennial favorite. In Bloomington, it was launched at us from the lips of young men with sunburnt shoulders, men who cruised town in battered trucks. Like so many four-letter words, its strong beginning and explosive ending gave it universal appeal. And so it was used by the suit-clad man in the expensive restaurant where we'd gone to celebrate our anniversary, the word slithering from his lips as we passed by, Mary in her crisply tailored suit jacket, me in my sleeveless summer dress.

"What did he say?" Mary asked, her voice growing thorns.

"Nothing," I demurred, grabbing her hand, leading her away. "He was talking to somebody else."

These moments made my stomach inch up into my throat and my eyes dart for escape. But my fears exasperated Mary, who'd made a name for herself studying rural queer life. Her research found that rural towns could be just as welcoming, if not more so, than big cities. But her academic research did not soothe my feelings of vulnerability.

An hour later we arrived at the Simon Cancer Center in downtown Indianapolis. Mary's hand steadied mine as we entered the lobby. Sunlight streamed through three stories of windows, energy charged the air. Behind the gleaming white information desk, a smiling face gave us directions to the breast center. Up a wide flight of stairs and to the left.

Entering the waiting room, my body relaxed. The ambiance was part spa, part library. The sunny space was arranged into several room-like divisions. Computers along one wall allowed patients to check email or surf the web while waiting. A small kitchenette had help-yourself tea, coffee, and light snacks. Past the check-in desk, a separate nook had reading chairs and a bookcase. On the bookcase were a series of binders, one for each doctor with plastic-sleeved pages holding a copy of the physician's CV, a personal statement about his or her approach to cancer care, and a list of authored publications. There were binders not only for the breast cancer surgeons but also plastic surgeons and radiation oncologists.

In the exam room, Cathy, Dr. B's nurse, did an intake. Her demeanor was warm and efficient, knowledgeable and caring. We told her we'd heard good things about Dr. B. She lowered her voice so as not to sound disloyal to the other surgeons in the practice. "He is absolutely the best surgeon we've got. You're in the right place."

A rustle in the hall produced a stout, bald man with frameless glasses and a walrus mustache. Apologies flew from his lips as he pumped my arm up and down and then pumped Mary's. He flipped through my file. The biopsy report came from where? St. Vincent's? "Well, we'll want to call them and request the slides so that we can retest the tissue," he said. "Our pathologists specialize in reading breast tissue biopsies, they are the best in the business."

Someone else to read and confirm the biopsy? Why hadn't I thought of that!

Mary made a note to call. I should explain that Mary was a speedy and studious scribe. If information was to be delivered during these appointments (and it always was), Mary was poised to receive it. Her background made her an expert at observing and recording human behavior, and my dealings with doctors and hospitals had become her informal field site. Eventually her handwriting—small, neat letters reminiscent of Campbell's Alphabet Soup—would fill several note-books with details of appointments, dates, times, diagnostics, and drug protocols. Her training kept her buckled into her logical, quick-thinking mind. For that I was grateful.

Grateful because I had checked out. In the weeks and months to come, friends would assume I—the women's health journalist—was steering my ship through breast cancer's choppy waters. They'd tell me how they envisioned me staying up late at night, my reporter's engines firing on all cylinders as I researched the latest treatments and downloaded peer-reviewed journal articles. While it was tempting to embrace this Hollywood montage version of myself, I had no energy for pretense, so I told them the truth. That the sheer force of my anxiety had blown my brain's fuse box early in the process. Whatever energy, thoughts, and consciousness that normally buzzed inside my cranium had gone dark, like blackout shades drawn in preparation for an air raid. My vision was fuzzy, my ears stuffed with cotton, the neurons of my brain glommed by fear. I fumbled through appointments with the stupor of someone who'd been concussed.

But my heart had stepped in to fill the void. I was a five-foot-four-inch living, breathing, walking heart. Not the red or pink ones you see on Valentine's Day or in children's drawings, but a bloody, pulsating expansion and contraction of tissue and fluids (mostly tears), sensitive to the slightest energies around me. Me-as-heart quivered, shook, and wept at the slightest provocation. A chirpy "How are you today?" from the speaker at the Starbucks drive-through was enough to choke me up. I'd never shied away from crying. Before cancer, I'd have a good cry every couple of weeks. After cancer, it was every couple of hours. The cancer diagnosis had shucked the shell right off my body.

On that morning in Indianapolis, Cathy stayed in the room, offering a distant but watchful presence during the physical exam. Dr. B's fingertips read my breast tissue and lymph nodes like Braille. Stopping. Starting. Interpreting. Digesting meaning. Of the three surgeons I'd seen, his touch was the surest, the most confident, the most thorough. He exuded expertise. Sensing his command of the situation, my shoulders loosened and the hinges of my jaw softened. Here was someone who'd dedicated his career to breast surgical oncology, someone whose job it was to teach others. Here, at last, was someone I could trust.

Dr. B stepped back and made his assessment. Like the two previous surgeons, he felt a lumpectomy with radiation was the answer, but the plastic surgeon would have the final say. Now I understood that the cancer surgeon's focus was on removing the cancer. Putting the breast back together was someone else's job.

Mary took notes as Dr. B told us about a new test to measure a tumor's aggressiveness called Oncotype. The results would take a couple of weeks, but he felt it was well worth doing as it would help inform future decisions, including chemotherapy and radiation. The same went for the BRCA1 and 2 tests. I liked that he was slowing down, gathering more information before rushing into surgery. I knew from the stories I'd written about breast cancer that the diagnosis was rarely a medical emergency. Because my tumor seemed to be slow-growing, another month wouldn't make a difference in my odds of survival, but careful planning might.

After Dr. B shook hands with us and left, Cathy gave me and Mary the room to discuss whether or not we wanted to move forward with scheduling the tests.

I told Mary how much I liked that Dr. B's practice was part of a larger hospital system. If I needed a scan, an ultrasound, or a procedure, it would all happen here. No driving between various medical offices. No syncing of medical records and insurance paperwork between providers. All things that would lower the odds of a mistake.

"Yeah," she said. "But he's a bit cocky, don't you think?"

A wave of annoyance rolled over me.

Why couldn't she just get onboard?

"He's a surgeon," I replied. "What do you expect? You'd have an ego too if you cut people open for a living."

"Okay. This is your decision. If you're sure, let's do it. Where do we sign up?"

With that I'd opened the third and final door of my Mystery Date. I'd made my match. But, knowing what I do now, I wish I'd given Mary's words more thought.

CHAPTER 7

From Indianapolis, zoom out, drag your eyes fifteen-hundred miles west across the country's waistband to Salt Lake City, Utah, where, at a molecular diagnostic company called Myriad Genetics, a machine was spinning a vial of my blue-red blood. What genetic secrets would it reveal? BRCA1? BRCA2? Was it you?

As we waited for results, urgency gave way to monotony. The lump adorned my chest like a broach. Insectlike, it burrowed under my skin, quietly nourishing itself, siphoning nutrients from my body. It drew my fingers like a magnet. Through the soft yarn of my sweater, through my bra underneath, I fiddled with cancer like it was a pebble in my pocket.

Before my diagnosis, Mary and I had planned a trip to Washington, DC. She had an academic conference, and I was going to spend the weekend with Beth and our new niece. But now I craved the comforts of home. Home bound me together, with the imprint of my pre-cancer self firmly embedded in its contours. Like my grandmother who relied on the familiar handholds—a countertop, a doorjamb, the post of a bed—to steer herself through her home of sixty years. I was feeble in a different way, dependent on my home's safe handholds—the dog, the brown couch, the garden—and the routines they enabled. The prospect of traveling to DC seemed risky, like releasing my hold on the ship's railing during a gale.

Our house had a first grader's love of right angles. A perfect rectangle with four large symmetrical windows—two on each floor—each window an eye with black shutters for lashes. The house was clad in white aluminum. A snaggletooth white picket fence hemmed the yard, which was roughly the same size as the home's modest footprint.

The interior was equally uninspired. The first floor had four rooms: living, dining, kitchen, and bath. The floor plan repeated upstairs with three small bedrooms and a second bath. We turned two of the bedrooms into offices. My office was twice the size of Mary's. I'd argued the extra space was necessary for yoga, and she didn't put up a fight. Mary is generous in ways I am not. She went on to paint her office a regretful cantaloupe hue. I painted mine the color of coffee ice cream. From my desk I had a view of the front yard, the rotting fence, and the intersection with its four-way stop. When I wasn't writing, I stared out the window. During the eight years in that house, I witnessed two fistfights, four fender benders, and dozens of stop-sign runners.

Mary and I had different experiences of home. My siblings and I had been raised to see property as an investment and rent as a waste of money. So much so that my older sister, Ginny, prided herself on having never paid a month of rent in her life. After college, she moved directly from the Peterson Palace into a red brick shotgun house of her own, securing the down payment with years of squirreled-away baby-sitting money. Although I had rented during my twenties, I'd also put away money from every paycheck for a down payment on a house of my own. By the time Mary got her job, I had ten thousand dollars in savings and the name of a mortgage broker.

Mary had grown up in a series of apartments and houses in Central California. Her single mother worked full-time and had little energy or spending money left for nesting. Rooms painted contractor beige stayed that way. Pictures were propped against walls, lest nail holes be subtracted from the deposit. Home was interchangeable and tempo-rary. Mary's Rolodex of childhood memories had no entry under trips to the paint store to choose a new shade of paint for her bedroom walls, no shopping for a bedspread to match, no jaunt to the frame store to place a poster or jigsaw puzzle under glass to hang on the wall for houseguests to admire.

Yet Mary knew I craved a home. A physical shell to anchor me in this world. A sense of ownership, of place, of control over my environment. A place where we could build a life and, hopefully, equity. More than anything, she wanted to make me happy, so a week after she got her job offer, we called a realtor.

The next weekend in Bloomington, the realtor drove us down quiet, leafy streets near the Indiana University campus. From the backseat of his SUV, Mary and I fawned over the rows of tidy Arts and Crafts bungalows with bountiful gardens and welcoming porches. But when the realtor looked at the numbers, it became clear that what we could afford was a "flip," a mile from campus in a neighborhood where pickup trucks on cement blocks doubled as lawn decor.

In the midst of the hunt, Mary went to San Diego to finish and defend her doctoral dissertation, a crucial step before starting her new job at the end of August. She was gone for a month. During her absence our realtor showed me the house on Rogers Street. Once a single-family home, the house had fallen into disrepair. For decades it was a cheap student rental. But a local contractor had bought it and was doing a gut reno. He'd offered my realtor and me a sneak peek. A few days later, as I picked my way through the skeleton-of-a-home, I saw potential in the hardwood floors, the plentiful windows, the claw-foot tub, and the substantial fireplace. My first-time-homebuyer eyes didn't see the contractor's shoddy workmanship or the bowing foundation. They saw sunny days, hot baths, and cozy fires. I sped to Kroger, bought a disposable camera, took twenty-four pictures, and returned to the one-hour photo counter. Later that evening as I hovered over his shoulder, the realtor scanned and emailed the photos to Mary in California. She called minutes later. "The bedrooms look kinda small, and did I see a four-way stop out front?" Her normally upbeat voice was starched with stress. "How busy is that street?"

"Trust me," I said. "The pictures don't do it justice."

"Okay, if it's really what you want."

I asked the realtor to draw up an offer. The house was ours before she got back. Within forty-eight hours of her return, we drove to Bloomington. Giddy with excitement, I took us through town, past the University, past the Kroger, turning left at the hospital, cresting a small hill, and there it was—our new home. I pulled to the curb and parked. We hopped out of the car and positioned ourselves across the street for a full view of our acquisition.

Nerves whisked at my stomach. The white aluminum siding was dingier than I'd remembered. The neighborhood shabbier. The street busier. As we stood in front of our house, a trio of men on Harley's braked hard at the intersection, a few feet from where we stood. For what felt like an eternity they revved their engines—VROOM, VROOM, VROOOOOM—before gunning toward town and leaving us in a cloud of diesel fumes. Mary hadn't spoken since we arrived. I glanced over at her and bit the edge of my lower lip. Was she going to say something? She remained silent. Her eyes locked on the eyes of the house, its lashes unblinking, its mouthlike door the color of blood. That's when I saw them—tears rolling down her cheeks.

When Mary reaches this telling of the story, she adds the things I miss. The parts about the crushing stress of morphing from a student into a professor within two weeks' time, about the pressures bundled into the job: publishing, class prep, and committee work. She will tell you that entering the job market at age thirty-four terrified her. She'd spent a lifetime accruing degrees, but all she could see was her empty bank account and looming student debt. She always said her only career goal was "to retire early," and she was panicked by her late start at saving for retirement. Unlike me, she hadn't grown up with the privilege of parents who could bail her out of financial emergencies, and what I didn't know was how much of her ambition—the momentum and drive I so admired—was fueled by fear. Fear that one misstep on the track toward academic success would send her spiraling into poverty.

Within two months of moving in, we discovered that while outwardly simplistic, the house was deft at masking its ailments. The seller had artfully disguised years of neglect—a new second-floor deck covered up the rotting roof beneath. New visible plumbing connected to plugged-up eighty-year-old pipes. And a two-story tree growing against the foundation, its eleven-inch diameter trunk enough to bow the foundation, was removed weeks before the house went on the market. The home inspector, a friend of the realtor's, identified the bowing foundation, which the contractor fixed, but he missed nearly everything else.

For the next five years, our relationship frayed and our savings dwindled as we shoveled money into the maw of home repairs. The basement needed floor-to-ceiling tuckpointing. The chimney needed rebuilding. The second-floor deck had to be torn off and rebuilt to staunch a cascade of water down the living room wall. And, finally, an expensive tree removal. Two thirty-foot water maples had towered over the house for decades. Now, one was dying. Remove it now or risk it falling on the house, advised the arborist. So, we emptied our bank account into his pocket and his crew dismembered the once majestic tree.

We'd started out as clueless caretakers, but over the years, we'd nursed the home back to health and in the process fallen in love with our hard-luck house. Now, after five years of work, the house felt familiar, known, safe. It belonged to us, and we to it.

That afternoon, Mary stood in my office, arms crossed, voice stern.

"We've got to make a decision about this trip to DC."

I sat at the helm of my smooth, white corner desk, a recent splurge after a banner year of freelancing. The desk was a weight anchoring me to my pre-cancer identity as a writer, a woman with a voice, a person with ambition beyond the next set of test results.

"You go. I'll stay here."

"Do you really think that's a good idea?" Mary rightly sensed that, if left alone, she'd return in three days to a chrysalis, shrink-wrapped in a cellophane of dark thoughts. "Why don't I cancel? The conference organizers will understand."

My stomach clenched. She'd skipped classes, missed department meetings, and requested extensions on deadlines. The least I could do was put my butt on a plane. So that weekend we flew to Washington, DC, and went our separate ways—her to the conference hotel and me to my little sister's house where the lump had new meaning.

Beth met me at her front door. Her heart-shaped face, curly hair, and freckles reminiscent of the toddler my seven-year-old self used to hoist onto her tiny hip to play mom. She opened her arms and we hugged on the threshold, our hearts saying all the words.

That night we sat in her living room on matching sage-green sofas, propped our feet up, and fell into our comforting rhythm of chatting and laughing. Competing to see who could crack the other one up. Caroline, whom I'd doted on all afternoon, was sleeping in her bassinet nearby. As the evening wore on, the baby began to mew. Beth scooped her up and returned with the baby in one arm and a nursing pillow in the other. Sitting down, she nestled the pillow around her waist, then laid the baby on top of it, like a gem. The four-month-old cooed and bicycled her chubby legs in anticipation. With one hand on the baby, Beth used her free hand to unzip her sweatshirt. She was still talking as she reached inside to unfasten her nursing bra. Then she stopped mid-sentence. Her hand froze. Her eyes darted around the room as if she'd forgotten to put something in place—the water bottle she always kept next to her while nursing or maybe the burping cloth?

"What is it?" I prompted, ready to be helpful. "Can I grab something for you?"

"Um."

"What?" I said.

"Should I go in the other room?" she asked. "I don't want to make you uncomfortable." Her eyes shifted toward the kitchen. "Maybe I'll just . . ." Her words trailed off as she pulled the baby tighter to her still-covered breast and started to get up.

Tears stung my eyes.

"Don't be silly!" I chortled, flapping my hand in her direction.

My little sister—the twelve-year-old I'd taught how to use a tampon, the teenager I'd inadvertently embarrassed with a copy of *Our Bodies, Ourselves* for her high school graduation, the woman whose hand I'd held in labor last fall—didn't want to breastfeed her newborn in front of me. She was afraid she would hurt my feelings. Afraid her breasts would remind me of what I stood to lose.

She settled back on the couch and began to breastfeed, cooing and smiling at her daughter.

Gathering my knees into my chest, I kept up my end of the conversation, swiping at tears when she wasn't looking. As the baby nursed, my shoulders curled in toward one another as if my body was circling its wagons against the inevitable.

Until that moment, I hadn't realized that my breast cancer could make other women feel uncomfortable about their intact bodies. What my sister didn't know and what I didn't have words to explain was that sharing intimate space with women was something I held dear. Maybe it was my years of single-sex education, maybe it was Osento, maybe it was a lesbian thing, but I found the relaxed mood of understanding and shared physicality among women deeply comforting. And, that night, sitting on my sister's couch, I felt it slipping away.

Later, lying in bed, listening to the house's unfamiliar nighttime noises—the furnace flickering on and off, the cat playing on the stairs, the neighbors in the adjoining townhouse—I played a new game called one in eight. Since one in eight women would be diagnosed with breast cancer during her lifetime, the game was that the person who got the disease could choose the next seven women to be spared. I compiled mental lists of women, starting with my sisters, my mother, Mary, and moving outward to include a rotating cast of friends and family members vying for those extra spots. As the weekend passed and I watched my sister fall deeper in love with her baby, no small part of me wished the game was real. My two sisters both had children. If one of the three of us had to go through breast cancer or—worst-case scenario, die—best it was me.

The next day, while my sister and the baby napped upstairs, I joined the cat in a sunny corner and pulled my book out of my shoulder bag. I'd packed *Dr. Susan Love's Breast Book*, thinking it would be good to re-familiarize myself with the basics. I'd never interviewed Dr. Love, but I'd used her book many times and found her a wise and trustworthy source. Sitting cross-legged in the sun room, light pouring in, I flipped through the chapter on risk factors. My eyes caught on a lone sentence standing, like an afterthought, at the bottom of the page. A sentence about radiation-induced breast cancer. About how women who had X-rays to monitor scoliosis during puberty were at increased risk. My stomach clenched. I snapped the book shut.

I'd suspected the radiation exposure I'd had in my early teens increased my risk, but it was another thing to see it spelled out in black-and-white as a scientific finding. Like many cancer patients, since my diagnosis, I'd panned the riverbed of my past for carcinogens. Mapped statistics, contemplated my risk factors. I found odd comfort in the uncontrollable ones, such as early menses. Women in my family got their periods young. I had been ten. Nothing to be done about it. But my gut lurched when it seized upon something controllable, something avoidable, like X-rays for a curve that hadn't troubled me until doctors suggested I try to fix it. Did too many X-rays during puberty cause my breast cancer? I'll never know. Cause and effect is rarely how cancer works, much less breast cancer. But I do suspect that the good intentions of well-meaning doctors have caused more suffering than anyone will ever know.

On my last night in town, Beth and I cleaned up after dinner. She loaded the dishwasher, I wiped down the counters. A knot tightened in the back of my throat. I'd been waiting to ask her something all weekend.

Voices drifted in from the television in the living room where my brother-in-law cradled the baby.

I chased cookie crumbs toward the sink with a wet paper towel then stopped next to Beth and took a quick breath. I had an early flight in the morning. It was now or never.

"Do you want to feel my lump?"

She froze. A fork in one hand and a yellow sponge in the other. Her narrow chin dropped, her right eyebrow arched—a trick she inherited from our father. Steaming hot water gurgled from the tap.

"If you've ever wondered, I mean, what it might feel like," I said.

I braced for a quick bite of sarcasm because that was how we rolled. But her features softened. Her eyebrow lowered. She crimped her forehead and nodded. Off went the water and down went the sponge. I guided her hand to my broach, my cancer pebble, my shard of glass. The one-in-eight game wasn't real, but this was something I could offer. An imprinting of knowledge through touch, the exquisite sensitivity of fingertips, gifted with the ability to distinguish self from other, to find a centimeter's worth of cancer in a sea of friendly tissue.

CHAPTER 8

Back at the IU Simon Cancer Center, Mary and I waited to meet the plastic surgeon, Dr. V. The exam room was small, windowless, and relentlessly beige. Sitting on the table, I shivered under the paper gown, thankful for the warmth of my jeans, wool socks, and winter boots.

In the corner, Mary colonized the hard plastic "guest" chair. She wiped her glasses clean and pulled her notebook and a thin black Sharpie out of her worn backpack. She'd come straight from class and still wore one of her teaching outfits—smooth gray pants and a burgundy sweater with a tailored dress shirt underneath, the cuffs neatly rolled up past her wrists. She ran her fingers through her bangs, brushing them away from her eyes. Her chestnut-brown hair was overgrown, almost long enough to tuck behind her ears. She glanced up at me and feigned a smile. "You ready for this?" she asked.

Before I could answer, the plastic surgeon's manicured hand swept the curtain back. He introduced himself with a bone-crushing grip and a blazing smile. He asked me to open my gown. I untied the string and faced him bare breasted. A WHOOSH of heat lit my face. Mary always teased me about my blushing. In the past two weeks, my body had been examined by many doctors, but Dr. V was the first who wasn't interested in the lump. He was looking at the size and shape of my breasts, a sculptor sizing up the quantity and quality of the raw materials.

Flames licked at my hairline.

My body shifted on the padded table and a small roll of belly fat heaved over the waistband of my jeans as if vying for the plastic surgeon's attention.

But his eyes stayed on my breasts. Would he notice the left was a smidgen bigger than the right? The day before, Mary had joked that a lumpectomy might even me out. "After all, leftie does have a little to spare."

More than once, Mary had called my breasts "the perfect handful," and I liked how well suited they were for my small frame. The size of peaches, they were unobtrusive enough for me to go bra-less under winter sweaters. And during the summer, a simple, minimally structured bra did the trick.

After what felt like forever, Dr. V drew the gown closed across my chest, a curtain falling on a stage.

"I'm afraid a lumpectomy is out of the question."

"Excuse me?"

Three surgeons—two breast surgeons and a general surgeon—had assured me a lumpectomy would take care of it. But the plastic surgeon, the person responsible for the end result, had the final say.

"A lumpectomy would decimate your breast."

The word *decimate* hung in the air between us.

Decimate sounded both vague and specific.

Hurricanes decimated coastal communities.

Earthquakes decimated cities.

There was no room in my neat-and-clean, worm-and-apple breast cancer metaphor for the word *decimate*.

A hollow space opened up behind my ribs, as if all the soft parts of my body had deflated like spent balloons. My breathing was shallow, my armpits slicked with sweat.

He explained that the location of my lump (high) and the size of my breast (small) meant I wasn't a candidate for a lumpectomy.

And just like that the most sensible and least-invasive treatment option was off the table.

He said a single mastectomy with reconstruction would be best. The reconstructive surgery best suited to my body was a latissimus flap, named for the back muscle (latissimus dorsi) that he would sever and use to fashion a new breast. He explained how he would carve apart the largest muscle in my back, and, with one end of the muscle connected to its blood supply, tunnel the loose end (the flap) through my body and under my arm until it reached the empty socket on my chest where my breast had been. Then he would pull the flap of muscle up and over a silicone implant. I pictured a steak laid over a tennis ball.

"Isn't that muscle doing something?" I asked.

"Most women hardly miss it," he said, his eyes on his notes.

Most women?

"Most women just want to look normal in clothes," he added, still not looking up.

Normal?

"You're not an athlete, are you?" At last, he glanced up from his clipboard.

I wanted to tell him about my yoga practice, how I'd spent years learning to trust my body's wisdom. Learning to overcome the quicksand of my fear. The real fear of falling. The irrational fear of snapping the metal rod that fused my lumbar spine. I wanted to tell him that yoga was where I'd made peace with my body. I wanted to tell him that my favorite pose was handstand, how I'd spent five years working up the confidence and the strength to put my hands on my mat and kick my legs to the sky. How hugging my upper back muscles into my vertical axis and balancing my weight on my hands made me feel strong and powerful in a world filled with messages telling me I was weak and in need of protection.

Instead, I answered, "Um, no, but . . ."

Just thinking about yoga had triggered my muscles to perk up, like Emma's ears when she heard the turn of the doorknob. My hands spread against the exam table, my shoulders lined up over my wrists, the wrapping of my outer shoulder muscles in and around my upper ribs. I knew without asking that headstands and handstands would be difficult, if not impossible, without my latissimus dorsi.

Dr. V explained how the skin of my chest could be stretched to make room for a breast implant. He'd wedge a tissue expander into the flat plane between my ribs and my chest muscle. Once a week for a few months, I'd visit his office where saline would slowly be injected into the inflatable device. As it expanded, it would tug, stretch, and coerce my chest muscle up and away from its moorings. Once the process was complete, he would operate to swap the tissue expander for an implant.

Goosebumps prickled up the backs of my arms. What would it feel like to have my pectoral muscle slowly ripped from its foundation? I pictured the KFC I'd eaten as a kid. The way my front teeth pulled the chicken's breast meat from the bone. The sound of its connective tissue tearing. The sight of those scrawny, matchstick-thin ribs underneath.

"Of course, matching a new breast to your existing breast is almost impossible." He explained that an implant would have a different shape and feel. "So we could put an implant in your other breast, too. You know, for symmetry. Insurance companies will usually cover surgery on the healthy breast, especially in women your age."

My mind raced to catch up. In less than an hour, my anticipated lumpectomy had escalated into two breast implants, a tissue expander, a harvested muscle from my back, and at least two surgeries, maybe more.

He paused.

Acid from my stomach sloshed at the base of my throat.

"Is there any other way? Something that doesn't involve implants and rearranging muscles?"

The question sounded childish. Why was I so peevish, so maladaptive that I couldn't get with the program?

Plus, there was another consideration. My scoliosis still caused my spine to curve, which meant my back was in a chronic state of torque and imbalance. Could it handle the loss of a key support beam? Was he even going to ask about pre-existing conditions? Prior surgeries?

A flood of panic rose in my lungs. The string of my hospital gown was wound around the tip of my index finger, and the skin had turned white.

Mary leaned forward in her chair, elbows on knees, her black notebook pressed between the cool of her palms. "Isn't there some other way?"

"Look," Dr. V said. He sighed, ran his hands through his hair, took a wider stance. The soles of his shoes squeaked on the linoleum. "If I do a lumpectomy, your breast will no longer look like a breast."

What about other reconstructive surgeries? Ones that used a woman's own tissue. Fat and muscle harvested from the belly, buttocks, or thighs, molded into a breastlike shape and grafted onto the chest. Native tissue looked more natural than an implant, and, unlike implants, it didn't need to be replaced. The downsides were significant. The surgery was much longer (six to seven hours) and the recovery much more painful, requiring several days in the intensive care unit and at least a week in the hospital.

"You're not a candidate for those procedures either," he said. "You are too thin. You don't have enough fat to make a new breast."

Did he just say I wasn't fat enough for a new breast?

Like most women, I'd been taught to equate thinness with femininity. Yes, I'd inherited my mother's high metabolism, but I kept one eye on my waistline. What woman hadn't? Now, Dr. V was telling me I was too thin for new breasts. By succeeding at one marker of femininity, I had positioned myself to fail at another.

My shoulders drew back.

"What if I didn't reconstruct?" I asked.

The final "t" sounded crisp and curt, more indicative of bravado than confidence.

I don't remember exactly how he answered me. But I do remember his inference that I'd be foolish to pass up the chance to get the breasts I'd "always wanted," as if all women pine for an upgrade.

An hour later, we were back in the car for the long drive home. Central Indiana's ceiling of soot-colored clouds flattened the midday light. We rode in silence. Me resting my temple against the window, seeking cold to balance out the exam room's sedating heat, which had left me numb and tired. Mary threading the car through downtown Indianapolis, past the art museum and the new Lucas Oil Stadium, and finally onto State Highway 37 south toward Bloomington.

Her hands rested at the responsible ten and two o'clock. My fingers plucked at the fabric of the car's upholstery.

At thirty-eight, was I ready to trust surgeons again? A lumpectomy was one thing, but the reconstructive surgery the plastic surgeon had proposed was invasive.

Could I trust him, with his blindingly white smile and youthful brown eyes, to rearrange my muscles?

Could I trust the companies that made the implants?

Even under the best circumstances, the Food and Drug Administration recommends that silicon implants be monitored with an MRI every two to three years to detect "silent leaks" and replaced roughly every ten years as the risk of rupture climbs with each passing year. Choosing implants would consign me to a lifetime of surgery, and each trip to the operating room would put me at risk of complications.

Years later I would learn that it's not unusual for breast reconstruction and its complications to send women to the operating room more than six times in the first two years. That one in three women who choose to reconstruct will have a major complication, such as an infection, and, in the case of tissue transfers, breakdown of the skin and death of the transferred tissue. But at the time, no one knew this yet, including the plastic surgeon, because the first comprehensive study to track and compare surgical outcomes of eight commonly used options for breast reconstruction surgeries, the Mastectomy Reconstruction Outcomes Consortium Study, wouldn't be funded for another three years.

The hum of the tires on wet pavement filled the car's interior like cotton batting. My mind scrambled for a fix, a way to achieve symmetry and balance. Into the thickness, I put the question to Mary. "What if I went flat?"

Her chin bobbed, a gesture that implied thoughtful consideration, but into which I read, "I'm stalling because I don't know what to say."

In hindsight, the question was a test. A pop quiz she would either pass or fail. Against her response I was set to weigh the substance of our ten-year relationship. How much did she love me? How much did she respect my autonomy? How much did she value my breasts? Was she willing to fight for them?

If anyone should have had a say about the future of my breasts, it was Mary. I loved her with this body. She loved me through this body. As a couple, we were long past physical infatuation. Clearly, she loved me for more than my breasts. But how could they not matter? Didn't she love me, at least in part, for my woman's body?

I didn't know it then, but what I needed was for Mary to pull over, cut the engine, take my hand in hers, tell me she loved my breasts—she'd be sad to see them go, but she'd support my decision no matter what. But her hands stayed on the wheel. The white winter sun glared off her silver wedding band. Our legal marriage was four years away, but we'd exchanged rings early on. Had we said the part about "in sickness and in health?" I couldn't remember.

Finally, we slowed to a stop at a red light in Martinsville, Indiana. Mary turned and put her hand on my knee. Her Justin Bieber bangs feathered across her forehead. A sly smile slid across her face. "You know I'm more of an ass man."

Mary always surprised me.

It was a spring night in 1998 when I stepped out of my apartment building onto the sidewalk of 18th Street in San Francisco's Mission District to go to a friend's "Ellen DeGeneres is coming out" party. Rumors had it that the comedian-turned-TV-star was going to come out on prime time that night, and the queer community was abuzz. A cold drizzle fell. To get my umbrella meant climbing up three flights of stairs and traipsing the long hallway to my tiny studio wedged in the back corner of the building. An incorrigible introvert, I knew if I got back up to my cozy room with its radiator heat, I'd never leave again, so I flipped the collar on my wool pea coat and plunged onward. The clang of the building's heavy iron gate still echoed in my ears as I rounded the corner and turned down Valencia Street.

A woman in a fire-engine red raincoat darted past. She exuded a sense of upbeat urgency. The buoyancy of her stride stood out among the neighborhood's slouching lesbians and sullen artists. Maybe she was from out of town. Seattle, most likely. People in San Francisco didn't wear red Gor-Tex. We were too hip for primary colors. As I walked up Valencia Street, I watched the red raincoat bob and weave. The raincoat hung a left on Twenty-Third Street. Same direction I was headed.

Were we going to the same party?

Who was she?

How did she walk so fast?

I cut the last corner onto Bartlett Street, and there she stood on the stoop of my friend's building, waiting for the telltale buzz and click that would signal the unlocking of the security gate. Rain seeped through the shoulders of the five-dollar coat I'd bought at Community Thrift, a neighborhood secondhand store. Maybe Gor-Tex wasn't such a bad investment after all.

When I reached the stoop, the woman broke into a crooked grin. Her red hood framed a round face, made even rounder by oval glasses and a pageboy bob. Freckles on her cheeks mirrored the raindrops on her glasses. The warmth and openness of her gaze took me aback. City people were standoffish. They didn't let down their guard until they knew exactly who you were and what you were about.

Didn't she know better than to trust me so quickly?

She stuck out her hand. "Hi, I'm Mary."

If you ask me, that night, standing on a sidewalk in the Mission, listening to the sound of tires on wet pavement, I fell in love. If you ask her, she'll tell you about our second encounter, a month later, at a birthday party for the same friend. In San Jose, at a Chinese restaurant, with fifty chatty women sitting around five round tables, Mary and I found one another and sat side by side. As the evening wore on, everyone and everything in the room slipped away until we were aware of nothing but each other.

Back in Bloomington after our meeting with the plastic surgeon, Emma met us at the door with joyful barks and wiggles. We turned on the floor lamps next to the couch and foozled the dog, but as soon as I went to scoop two cups of kibble into Emma's dinner bowl Mary retreated to her office to hole up for the rest of the night and work.

My editors had extended my deadlines. The world of magazines was different than the world of academia. Mary was closing in on tenure and any delay would be considered a sign of weakness, a wavering of her commitment to the University. I was jealous of her ability to concentrate on work even though later she would tell me she was anything but focused. Still, for Mary, work appeared to be a convenient escape, an all-consuming taskmaster. With no such mental safe place, I set about making a physical one.

Our house had two bathrooms. The downstairs bathroom was the more spacious of the two, big enough for a six-foot-long, cast-iron claw-foot tub. Five years ago, the tub had sold me on the house. Although the walls were still stripped to the studs, the tub's weight and solidity anchored the downstairs bathroom, helping me see past the flotsam of construction and toward a future filled with candlelit soaks.

After we moved in, that's exactly what I did. On most nights, you could find me in the tub, particularly in the winter when a hot soak was the only way to shake the damp Midwestern cold. Every evening, when Mary slipped upstairs into her office, I'd stuff the cracked plug into the tub's rusty drain, turn the water spigot on full blast, and empty out the contents of our fifty-gallon hot water tank.

The claw-foot tub in our Indiana house reminded me of the Peterson Palace. My parents' house had five bedrooms, one for them and one for each of us four kids. Three of the bedrooms were on the second floor—one for my parents, one for my younger sister, and one for my brother. The other two bedrooms and a small bath were on the house's third floor, accessed from a cramped stairway at the back of the house. Rumor had it that the third floor had once been a ballroom, and I liked to imagine women in satin and chiffon gowns twirling across the hardwood floor instead of the cavernous room spliced down the middle by a temporary wall my parents had erected. This was where my older sister, Ginny, and I would sleep until we left for college.

Off the third floor's short hallway was an afterthought of a bathroom. To enter, you took an awkward step up, followed by a sharp right. The walls and ceiling were coated in cracked paint the color of toenail fungus. A bare lightbulb dangled on a black cord over the rust-stained pedestal sink. The long, thin bathroom was the size of a pipsqueak bowling alley, yet, somehow, it held a black, full-sized, cast-iron claw-foot tub. To imagine the tub's journey into the house—up the grand central staircase, down the second floor's narrow hall, and up the skinny stairwell to the third floor—was as much a wonder to my child's eye as the building of the pyramids. Yet, there it sat, an elephant in a shoebox.

Because the bathroom was functional, it went untouched for years. Decades of deferred maintenance had left my parents with more pressing concerns to address, such as the house's crumbling chimneys, rotting porches, and a roof with more leaks than my mother had pots. But then one day it was time to renovate the decrepit bathroom by opening it up.

After years of utilitarian house repairs, my mother's blue-gray eyes sparkled with her vision of a pink-and-white bathroom. A bookish, independent woman, she had an eye for interior decorating, and pastels were her preferred palette. A few weeks later, Ginny and I came home from high school to find the room doubled in size. Next came drywall and a new vanity. Then came a wallpaper hanger to cover an accent wall with a floral print—a white background with green curlicue vines and cotton candy–pink flowers. My mother painted the other walls bubblegum pink.

As the bathroom's final flourish, my mother painted the black claw-foot tub a high-gloss white. On the last day of her grand design, the woman who scoffed at girly things like manicures and makeup gave the ancient tub a dainty pedicure. I can picture my mother on her hands and knees, dipping a teeny craft paintbrush into the leftover gallon of pink paint and delicately tracing the brush over the nails on each of the tub's four clawed feet. She'd be wearing her paint-spattered blue Oxford cloth shirt over one of our old Camp Earl Wallace T-shirts. Her socks bunched at her ankles. Drugstore slippers or cracked, brown leather loafers on her feet. She'd bite her lower lip and squint at the tub's toenails, wanting to stay inside the lines. The bathroom renovation was a radical improvement, and my older sister and I took the girly flourishes in stride. We were inured to my mother's approach to femininity—she dabbled in it but she didn't take it too seriously.

Now, as a grown woman with my own money-pit house and my own seen-better-days claw-foot tub, I dribbled lavender-infused bath oil across the water's steaming surface. To ease myself into the tub, I clamped my hands around the cool, cast-iron lip and lowered myself slowly, an inch at a time, until—a half-dozen sharp, short inhales later—my body slipped beneath the surface. During these long winter baths while I lay in the tub's smooth embrace, a simple white washcloth kept my breasts warm. A clean washcloth, trailed through the hot water and draped across my half-submerged breasts. Candlelight flickering, lavender-laced steam rising. Eyelids fluttering closed, body suspended and relaxed, adrift between two worlds. Every few minutes, I'd pinch the top two corners of the cloth, peel it off, trail it under the water to reheat, and draw it back up across the chest. An intuitive gesture performed countless times.

But, in the shadow of my cancer diagnosis, baths took on new meaning. Lying in the tub, I saw my body through a new lens. The lump had been growing for ten years. What else was it hiding? Many of the women in online breast cancer support groups were angry at their bodies, using words like *betrayal* to describe them. But betrayal sounded too intentional to my ear, too much like a choice or a moral failing. My friend Patricia had offered me an alternative, suggesting that solid tumors were, in part, capsules the body makes to protect itself. Whether or not it was true, I wanted to give my body the benefit of the doubt, imagining it building a wall around the rogue cells, like surrounding a barrel of nuclear waste in concrete, more symbolic than effective, but a good effort all the same.

That night, after the consult with the plastic surgeon, as I relaxed into the tub, a hollowness opened at the back of my throat. My fingertips traced the satiny scar of my back surgery, a thin, white ribbon running the length of my left side, from shoulder to hip. Picture twelve-year-old me, wanting her parents' attention and agreeing to an unnecessary spinal fusion because she didn't know there were other options.

Now picture thirty-eight-year-old me. She deeply understands that she is the one who must live inside this body. Live day-in and day-out with her decision after the doctors have all moved on. She knows happiness rests on her ability to be in her body freely, without pain. Without restriction. She wonders if she has grown into the advocate her younger self needed.

CHAPTER 9

The following afternoon, hunched at my white desk, I moused over to Amazon to order a breast cancer book a friend had recommended, and lo and behold there was an espresso machine in my cart. My hand stopped midclick. Where did that . . . ? Oh, right. Last time I'd visited the site, it was to buy myself a late-Christmas present. I'd spent hours online comparing prices and brands. Now, in early February, that person—a woman who'd cared about finding the perfect espresso machine—was gone. I realized she had no idea how carefree her life had been. How she'd taken for granted that her future was stretched out in front of her, that she'd live to see her nieces and nephews grow up, that she'd be around to enjoy the retirement fund she and Mary contributed to every month. I punched the delete button next to the coffeemaker. Today I had no time or money for espresso. This month's decision was whether or not to amputate one breast or two, to reconstruct or not to reconstruct.

Yesterday the plastic surgeon made it clear that my breast was too small for a lumpectomy. I hadn't even known that was possible. He'd explained that a mastectomy was the only way forward. My only decision, he said, was how I'd like to reconstruct. Up until two weeks ago, no man had ever touched my breasts, and now both the plastic surgeon, Dr. V, and the breast cancer surgeon, Dr. B, seemed very concerned about their well-being.

I loved my breasts. And I loved having breasts. Breasts made me feel feminine and soft, curvy and desirable. What was I willing to put my body through to keep some semblance of breasts? Was a muscle laid over an implant enough? The plastic surgeon had been clear that it would look less like a breast and more like a "breast-shaped mound."

My fingers tapped the white and silver keyboard. A Google search brought up hundreds of pre- and post-mastectomy photos. The greatest number of photos were on plastic surgeons' websites—photos of women who'd undergone reconstruction after breast cancer, photos cropped to protect the patient's identity.

Yesterday, in the doctor's office, the surgeon's words "breast-shaped mound" sounded odd, but in looking at these photos, it was clear the phrase was not hyperbolic. The pictures of reconstructed breasts were indeed mounds of tissue or, in some cases, a mashup of an implant covered by tissue taken from other parts of the body. The mounds reminded me of Jello-molds, unnaturally stiff and uniform in the way they sat on women's chests. I could imagine a reconstructed breast would look more natural when concealed by clothing. But that begged the question: Who was I fooling? What I loved most about having breasts was less about how they looked in clothes and more about the pleasure they brought to the bedroom. If I were to reconstruct, my breast-shaped mound would have no nipple and no feeling. The pleasure of this reconstruction would not be mine.

I was struck by how little I understood about the logistics of breast reconstruction. For years, women's magazines had paid me to write about lumpectomies and mastectomies. I'd talked to women on both sides. I'd interviewed plastic surgeons who specialized in breast reconstruction. But clearly my questions had fallen short. I'd assumed breast reconstruction was much like breast augmentation. Now it's clear that one surgery enhances breast tissue while the other removes it. In an augmented breast, the implant nestles under the breast tissue like a baseball into a catcher's mitt. In a post-mastectomy breast, no breast tissue could be left behind to soften or conceal the implant because of the risk of recurrence, so surgeons are forced to get more creative.

But there was another thing: in truth, most of my editors wouldn't have been interested in a reconstruction-after-breast-cancer story. These women at the helm of publishing (and they were mostly women) assigned single-note breast cancer stories. Reflecting the culture at large, they preferred chirpy, feel-good articles about mammograms saving lives, pink ribbon charities funding a cure, and survivors thankful for breast cancer's wake-up call. Inside the pages of these magazines, breast cancer was often portrayed as a minor inconvenience. Editors were also at the mercy of advertisers. Companies didn't want their products displayed next to stories about complications, painful surgeries, and implants that ruptured or hardened with scar tissue. For all the lip service women's magazines had given breast cancer, for all the money they'd made selling advertising to companies who slapped pink ribbons on everything from cars to mixers, no one cared about preparing women for the reality of the disease. Or maybe it's more accurate to say there was no bright-siding that message, so it was easy to ignore.

Another question nagged at me: How complicit had I been in the erasure of the truth about breast cancer?

I stared out the window at the remaining maple tree in our yard, its straight trunk and strong branches stark against the winter backdrop.

The phone rang. It was my mother. My guess was she wouldn't have thought twice about giving up her breasts. I imagined she'd say they'd served their purpose. She'd breastfed four babies and now she'd be happy to be rid of them. She was nothing if not stoic. She considered unpleasant emotions a waste of time. "Just get over it," she'd chime to our girlhood tears. My sisters and I became the keepers of one another's emotional lives. As we got older, we told ourselves that Mom was just a product of her generation, one that made do without making a fuss. The "suck-it-up generation." But as I got older I tried to take chances with her, to open the door to connection, even if she chose not to walk through it.

"I've been surfing plastic surgery websites looking at before-and-after pictures of breast cancer surgeries," I told her. "I'm feeling torn about what to do."

Could I hear her shrug over the phone or was it my imagination?

"Why don't you just do what Bonnie Collins did and stuff socks in your bra?"

"Excuse me?"

Bonnie had been my mother's best friend for thirty years and was a fixture in our family. She was fiercely intelligent and wickedly funny. The wife of a politician and the daughter of a well-heeled Southern family, the kind my grandmother might call "high cotton."

"What are you talking about?"

"Bonnie stuffed her bra with old nylons and socks after her double mastectomy."

"Whoa, what?"

Bonnie and my mother shared season tickets to the Louisville Ballet. Once a month, on a Friday evening, she'd materialize in our house like Glenda the Good Witch, floating through the back door and into the kitchen on a cloud of perfume. Us kids would be sitting at the table spooning mac and cheese into our mouths, my mom getting ready upstairs, and we'd stare at Bonnie's silk blouse and pearl necklace. My face was level with her substantial bosom. To my child's eyes, Bonnie's torpedo-shaped breasts had been a thing of wonder.

"When you guys were little," my mom said, "you wouldn't remember but her mother died of breast cancer, and Bonnie had hers lobbed off right then and there. Her bra has been nothing but socks ever since."

The admiration in my mother's voice was palpable. She approved of women who made the best of a bad situation and didn't complain.

Wait, Bonnie's breasts were fake? She was flat?

The sound of water running in my mother's kitchen sink thundered in my ears. Always practical, she liked to do the dishes while talking on the phone. The phone's putty-colored base was mounted on the brick wall next to the kitchen sink. I pictured her up to her elbows in banana-yellow rubber gloves, her right shoulder hitched up to hold the receiver to her ear, the vise grip of her cheek the only thing saving the phone from plunging into the soapy water.

"Can I call you back?"

"Sure thing."

I hung up, thinking of all the times Bonnie Collins had swirled into our house, how she had offered me a version of womanhood different than my mother's. My mother dressed up for the ballet, too, but even in a brocade suit, nylons, and wedge heels, her nonconformist nature was evident in her hands calloused from gardening, her fingernails pruned for practicality, and her cheeks ruddy from wind and sun. It was Bonnie who relished her mascara, her manicure, and her ivory satin headband.

Had I really grown up within arm's length of a breastless woman and not even known!

How might I be different today had I known just one woman who'd laid claim to her post-mastectomy body? A woman who'd made her flatness visible?

How many other women in my adolescent landscape had a similar secret?

How I hated secrets! I'm seven years old. It's the Saturday morning before Christmas, and my siblings are poring over the Sears Wish Book making lists of the gifts they want from Santa. My older sister wants a Star Wars X-wing fighter. My brother wants a Tonka semi-trailer truck with detachable cab. My bullshit meter is running high, so I creep into my parents' bedroom where my father is fast asleep. Sleep is precious to him. He despises being woken up, especially on weekends, but it's worth the risk—the truth is at stake. I scramble up onto the mattress, straddle his mountain of a stomach, and begin demanding he tell me the truth about Santa Claus.

"You wouldn't lie to me, would you Dad?" I said in my most-inno-cent-little-girl voice.

He laughed.

"Do you really want to know?"

His voice was somber, which told me he was serious.

I nodded. He made me promise not to tell my siblings.

Outside the window the sky was turning rose-petal pink. Mary would be home soon. A pang registered in the hollowness of my gut. Mary and I had chosen not to have kids of our own but we had enough nieces and nephews to make a basketball team, and we wanted to be as open and honest with them as possible. When they were little, I'd welcomed their questions about my girlish clothes and boyish hair, about my painted toenails and unshaven legs. There would be no pretending, no dodging questions. Confidence didn't always come easily, especially when I'd see one of the little ones sizing me up from across the room, puzzling which camp to put me in: blue for boys or pink for girls. But Mary and I wanted to be ourselves in front of them.

We thought about the kid question long and hard. When we first toured our house in Bloomington, the realtor described the small upstairs room as "the perfect size for a nursery." Like many people, he'd assumed that two women, with biological clocks ticking in tandem, would be bursting with maternal desire. We'd considered kids (what lesbian couple hadn't?), but between our late career start and the expense, our conversations always ended on an ambivalent note. As time went on, we got to know ourselves better. Mary was more devoted to work than either of us realized at first, and my thirst for a hermitlike solitude was strong. Eventually, we knew we'd make better aunts than parents. So, the room became her office.

I flipped on my desk light. My eyes burned from hours in front of the screen. The hinges on my office door creaked as Emma's Milk-Dud nose wedged the door open. She planted herself in the doorway, her hitched-up eyebrows saying *dinnertime*. I swiveled back to the screen. A sigh and a series of soft thumps meant she'd settled on the floor to wait.

"Just a few more minutes," I told her as my fingers curled around the mouse. Page after page of breast-reconstruction surgery scrolled past. "Somewhere in here, there's gotta be someone like me."

The next night, swimming through the crowded yoga studio, heat and humidity enveloped me like a blanket. The floor was a sea of young women with taut bellies, toned limbs, and perky breasts. They lazed in various postures of repose, reclined on their mats as if glitterati at a Hollywood pool party. I tiptoed between their pink and purple mats, trying not to trip over Evian bottles or Lululemon hoodies.

Old me was allergic to fitness-focused yoga classes, finding them vapid and vain. She was drawn to yoga for its calm, meditative side. But new me was all about getting strong before surgery in hopes of a speedy recovery. She didn't have time for meditation. Vapid and vain was exactly what new me needed. Besides, Lucy, the studio owner, had invited me to binge on as many classes as I could, free of charge—and nothing got me out of the house like a freebie. That's how, on a frigid night in late February, I found myself in a class billed as "hot fusion," a blend of yoga poses and lifting free weights in a room heated to over one hundred degrees.

I'd discovered yoga a month after I moved to San Francisco. I'd just turned twenty-six. I was walking up Sixteenth Street in the Castro, a neighborhood where Victorians were wedged together as tightly as books on a shelf. The setting sun glowed behind Twin Peaks, the air electric with the heady energy of a completed workday. My eye caught on a brightly painted door. Next to the door was a window with a simple white curtain through which a peaceful yellow lamp glowed. A handwritten sign listed a few yoga classes and named the studio as The Blue Door. I went back the next night, and the next, and the next.

The teacher's name was Wendi, and for the next five years she taught me how to listen to my body. She had me line up my hands and feet along the square pattern of the stick-on linoleum in the converted basement-turned-studio. Simple poses: triangle, tree, boat. Every pose an awakening. She taught me how to do yoga from the inside out, how to enter the stillness, how to read my body's patterns of holding, how to coax it into releasing and realigning. Yoga became my entry into a deep, quiet, introspective space and sparked a lifelong curiosity. My back aches all but vanished. Six years after my first class, I became a yoga teacher. I specialized in yoga for healthy backs. For eight years, I offered a weekly yoga class in Bloomington.

The class I was attending today was not that. Since those early days, the nation's yoga boom had transformed the practice into a homogenous, hyper-feminine space where the price of admission was one-hundred-dollar tights, a ponytail, and a BMI of less than 18.5 percent. My heart broke a little thinking about how my awkward, hairy, queer twenty-six-year-old-self would never have dared to cross the threshold of a yoga studio if the students looked like the ones in the room tonight.

For the next hour, Lucy's voice guided us through sun salutations and standing poses. My body moved through the motions while my mind made lists of questions:

What was harder: The idea of losing my breasts or the idea of reconstructing them?

Would a prosthesis mean I'd need to wear a bra to look balanced?

Would it shift when I reached my arm overhead?

What about swimming?

Would I need a second, waterproof breast for the beach?

Here is one thing I knew: I craved ease in my body. Simple things like being able to wake up, slip on a T-shirt, and take Emma for a walk without fussing with a bra and prosthesis. Kicking up into a handstand during yoga without worrying that my fake boob might plop to the floor.

On the spectrum of "body parts I could live without," where did my breasts fall? Surely they were less important than an arm or a leg? But what about my little toe or a pinky finger?

Here's another known: breasts were a big part of sex for me. A light pinch or nibble from Mary was enough to get me aroused. When we were making love, I'd let my nipples skim the sensitive skin of her stomach as I kissed her breasts.

But if I had one breast missing would sex be the same?

Would fear of a recurrence poison my tender feelings toward the remainder?

In my remaining breast would I see only the possibility of another cancer?

Beyond sex, what value did my breast hold? I had no need to attract a husband or nourish babies. My breasts served no practical measure beyond filling out a dart in a dress.

As the class wore on, my body felt lighter, more aligned. I should explain that being in my body is like driving a car with a steering wheel that pulls to the left. Scoliosis makes me drift off center. My left side is stronger than my right. The strength translates to larger muscles that are more contracted, more likely to spasm or seize. When that happens, my vertebrae are quick to jump the rails, which sends me straight to the chiropractor. I am careful not to aggravate my lopsidedness. I don't bowl. I don't play tennis. I don't carry a heavy shoulder bag. But yoga's emphasis on stretching and strengthening both sides evenly nudges my body toward strength and balance. All of this is to say that I didn't know how I would handle the asymmetry of one breast.

Would I be distracted by a nagging feeling of unevenness?

If I chose a single mastectomy with reconstruction, would the reconstructed breast weigh more than my natural breast, leaving me off balance?

Choosing an implant or to be one-breasted would create a permanent imbalance. If the curve in my back responded poorly to the shift in weight, no chiropractor or yoga class would be able to undo it.

After class, the lights came up and the young women rolled their mats, blotted their glistening foreheads, and smoothed back wisps of hair that had escaped their blonde ponytails.

CHAPTER 10

In the five weeks between diagnosis and surgery, craving the companionship of women who'd been pressed into this choice, I spent hours online clicking and scrolling through breast cancer community forums. The forums drew thousands of patients, primarily women, who commiserated about everything from treatment regimens, such as chemo cocktails and tips on how to soothe radiation burns; to logistics, such as how to arrange child care during hospital stays. Skimming for surgery threads, I found dozens of ongoing conversations about reconstruction. Women cheered each other on through eight-hour surgeries, multiple infections, and months of recuperation. Everyone was making lemonade out of their diagnosis and opting for new boobs.

Hyperlinks sent me to plastic surgery sites where women's bodies were covered with dotted lines to show tissue that would be harvested to make new breasts. These were "flap" surgeries where surgeons took a woman's own skin, fat, and sometimes muscle, and moved it to her chest to fashion a breast-shaped mound. Most often, tissue came from the lower abdomen, the inner thigh, and the buttocks. In the pictures, the dotted lines on women's bodies looked like the "cut here" lines on paper dolls. The soft roll of a woman's belly, the generous curve of her thigh translated into a breast waiting to happen. As if women's bodies came with a spare breast, like a spare tire for a car.

Plastic surgeons seemed to view a woman's body as a collection of parts to be disassembled and reassembled according to the cultural construct of femininity. Belly fat = bad. Breasts = good. Solve two problems at once. The procedure where belly fat is repurposed into a breast, a DIEP flap, is even called a tummy tuck reconstruction. All of this makes sense in a culture where breasts are seen as a measure of a woman's worth. Where being feminine is synonymous with being desired by men.

Clearly, I was out of step. I was a nonconformist by nature, but not seeing myself reflected in this world felt shitty nonetheless. I'd been diagnosed with the womanliest and pinkest of cancers, and I wasn't fitting in with my peer group. I didn't want to sacrifice a muscle to rebuild my breast, and I felt alone in valuing the structural integrity of my body, the beauty of its operating system.

A double mastectomy was not a get-out-of-cancer-free card. It would not lower my odds of dying from breast cancer. Women who've had double mastectomies die from the disease just as often as women who've chosen lumpectomy, reconstruction, or some combination of the above. But a double mastectomy would lower my odds of a breast cancer recurrence. That meant something to me. I didn't want to go through this again. Plus, if it came back, my cancer would be more aggressively treated. One breast cancer diagnosis was bad luck. Two was a tragedy.

My disorientation was not assuaged by my doctors who seemingly worried about the fate of my breast as much as they fretted over my cancer. To occupy such a terrifying moment and realize that the people who'd come to save me weren't seeing me but seeing their projection of a woman, a one-dimensional paper doll, with a breast in need of saving was confusing at best and terrifying at worst.

Later that week, my friend Tad came by the house and we spirited ourselves upstairs and into the bedroom. Tad was transgender and raised female. He'd undergone top surgery years before. What had prompted each of us to consider surgery was very different, but he was the only person my age who'd had a double mastectomy without reconstructed breasts.

His fingers fumbled with the buttons on his navy-blue shirt. I kept one eye on the bedroom door, not wanting Emma to bust it open and leave him feeling exposed and vulnerable. My stomach twitched as if we were two scheming teenagers. A few seconds later, the last button slipped out and he opened his shirt to reveal a white cotton undershirt. He removed the button-down, hanging it by the collar on the door-knob. He stopped to clear his throat.

Ugh. Was this too much to ask? Would this damage our friendship?

He and I were alike in that we were both shy and sensitive. But there was so much I'd never know about the years of pain and anguish he'd gone through to become who he was today. What I did know was that he was kind and generous, if not a bit cranky, like me. He was also a studious consumer of health care. Like most queer-identified trans men, he had to be careful. Seeking out surgeons and providers who were able to open their minds beyond the binary.

For my part, I'd just spent days scrolling through pictures of cookie-cutter implants and breast mounds crafted from flaps of tissue. I wanted to know what a reconstructed flat chest looked like when a surgeon applied the same skill and care that so many plastic surgeons were applying to reconstructed breasts.

Sitting on the bed, my hands shoved under my thighs, I stared at Tad's thick-soled work boots, then lifted my gaze up past his slim waist just as his fingers took hold of the hem of his white undershirt and lifted it. An appreciative "whoa" was all I could muster. The skin of his chest was flat and smooth. He had small, round nipples, each one centered on top of a plateau of pec muscle. There were no glaring scars. No bumpy outcroppings of ribs. No "dog ears" caused by the extra flaps of skin some surgeons left behind at the incisions' outer edges.

He showed me where his surgeon had hidden the scars in the grooves beneath the pec muscles. What? Every mastectomy photo I saw had a thick scar that ran straight across the middle of the breast, as if the surgeon was slicing open a baked potato. All of the flap surgeries left massive scars. There was no attempt to hide anything. But Tad's scars were barely visible, hidden in the shallow dip between his chest and upper abdominal muscles, two thin pencil lines.

The part of me that is versed in sexuality and gender 101 knows there is no comparison between a transgender man's post-op chest and a cisgendered woman's double mastectomy after a breast cancer diagnosis. But the part of me that was freaking the fuck out about what my own chest was going to look like at the end of this ordeal was the part that was in the bedroom with Tad that afternoon, the part that had mustered the confidence to ask such a personal favor. And the latitude I had to explore these questions was shaped and enabled by queerness.

The beauty of queer culture was the diversity and plurality of its citizens and their intimacies. Being queer meant pushing against cultural assumptions of who you are supposed to love and what bodies are meant to look like. It was a provocation to do things differently. When my doctors told me I should reconstruct my breasts, they were coming from a place I'd abandoned long ago—a place where it was important for women to have breasts because breasts were desirable to men. Because I didn't want to be desired by men, I had the freedom to explore what I wanted for myself.

A week later, Mary and I went to my appointment with Dr. B, the breast cancer surgeon. Mary had a new notebook and a list of follow-up questions. I had the image of Tad's chest emblazoned on my brain. When Dr. B asked if I had any questions about the surgery, I launched into a description of Tad's chest, how his surgeon hadn't cut straight across the midline of the breast but instead had hidden the incisions at the bottom of the pec muscle. I described how Tad's chest was flat but shapely, not like the pictures of mastectomies I'd seen online.

Dr. B raised an eyebrow. He brought two fingers to his upper lip and made a wide O with his mouth as he drew them along the either side of his mustache, smoothing it down.

Mary's expression darkened.

Words tumbled from me, falling in a heap on the floor. "You couldn't even see his scars, they were hidden right here." I drew a line with the tip of my index finger underneath my breast.

Dr. B cleared his throat.

"You have cancer. Cancer surgery is different."

My heart sank.

"There is a protocol," he said. "The scar will be across the middle. That's how I do all of my mastectomies."

I felt like a fussy diner who'd tried to order off the menu.

"Is there any way to save my nipples?"

"No. That's not an option. The nipples contain breast tissue, they can't be spared."

My choices were full-on breast reconstruction or straight-up mastectomy.

A few minutes later, Cathy came into the room. Good news, she said, there was an opening in the surgery schedule next week at a satellite hospital in Martinsville, a small town only twenty minutes outside of Bloomington. She told us how Dr. B had established the hospital's breast surgery center the year before, and he operated there every Tuesday. She assured us that the quality of care would be the same and reminded us that it would be more convenient because it was so much closer to our house.

My mouth opened, then closed. I glanced at Mary knowing she would have the words to explain our hesitation. Martinsville had a reputation for being one of the most conservative towns in Indiana. Recently, it was in the news for having hosted a Ku Klux Klan rally. Every Halloween, the mega-church hosted a "Hell House," an attraction similar to a haunted house, but instead of ghosts and goblins, the house was filled with sinners. A key component of such houses was a roomful of people dying of AIDS because they'd sinned against God for having sex with men.

"We were under the impression that Martinsville might not be, well, the most open-minded place," Mary said.

Cathy's eyes toggled from Mary to me and back to Mary. "I can't imagine it'll be a problem," she said. "But I've got a friend who's a nurse down there. Let me give her a call and I'll be right back."

Not until 2015, six years later, would Federal law recognize all LGBTQ marriages and ensure same-sex couples the same rights to visit one another in the hospital that straight couples enjoyed. Had something terrible happened during or after my breast cancer surgery, Mary could have been prevented from seeing me and making any decisions about my care, even though, like many same-sex couples we knew, we'd had legal paperwork drawn up for just such an occasion. We'd printed it out, folded it into a manila envelope, and carried it in the glove compartment of our car in case we were ever in an accident and one of us was badly injured. The multi-page document said, in essence, that we were family. Even so, we knew that legal paperwork was flimsy at best. Friends' experiences had taught us that encountering one homophobic gatekeeper at a hospital who refused to recognize the document was all it took to erase the safeguards queer couples so carefully tried to construct.

Ten minutes later, Cathy came back in the room. Her eyes were downcast. "Yes. Um. About Martinsville . . . I'm sorry to say we'll need to do your surgery here in Indianapolis after all."

The next day, Mary and I took Emma on a long dog walk through the leafy neighborhood between our house and the campus. Mary held the soft leather of the well-oiled leash. She listened and nodded as I ran through my options, listing the pros and cons. Usually she was quick to add her own thoughts, showing me what my argument was missing, helping me see things from her perspective. But she was unusually quiet. She was giving me room to try on different ideas, to come to my own conclusions. Her support was palpable, but she knew whether or not to reconstruct had to be my decision.

Later that day, while on the phone with a close friend, came the question I knew many of my friends were wondering: "But why would you want to remove them both?" A wave of defensiveness rose in my chest. I wanted to snap at her, tell her she wouldn't understand, she'd never had cancer, she'd never had to contemplate amputating one breast or two.

She brought up a headline she'd seen in the *New York Times* about the rise in breast cancer patients opting for double mastectomies. Like me, the majority of women making this choice were younger, white, and well educated. The articles quoted doctors who were flummoxed at why women were choosing prophylactic removal of their healthy breast as well as the cancerous one. To be clear, unlike me, most of these women were reconstructing both breasts. But, either way, more women were choosing to remove two breasts instead of just one. Even women who, unlike me, were candidates for lumpectomy.

I took a deep breath. Clearly, many women handled a single mastectomy with grace, but I didn't see myself as one of them. I shuddered at the prospect of feeling even more lopsided in my off-kilter body. I felt stymied by the logistics of corralling a singleton in a world built for two. And, if I'd reconstructed, my breast-shaped mound would have no feeling. As I aged, the implanted breast wouldn't droop like my bio-breast, meaning I'd be asymmetrical. And then there would be the heavy monitoring of my so-called healthy breast that would forever shackle me to a mammography machine and its attending anxieties.

She let out an exacerbated "harrumph."

I knew I hadn't changed her mind, but I had clarified my own.

"Have you gathered your tribe?" asked Patricia the week before surgery. She lived in Boulder, Colorado, and her cancer treatment had just ended. She was twenty years older than me and one of my only friends who knew what it was like to be diagnosed with cancer. Like me, she ate organic, exercised, and was tuned into her body. And, like me, she often had people respond to news of her disease by saying, "How can you have cancer? You're the healthiest person I know!" I never knew what to say to people in that moment. The moment when my situation didn't align with their idea of me. Or their idea of who was supposed to get cancer.

"What?" I asked, unable to hide my distaste for the hippy-dippy sound of the word *tribe*.

"You know, your people, your friends, you need to call on people for support. Don't go this alone."

"I'm not alone. I have Mary," I said.

"Right. How's she holding up?"

"Okay," I lied. What I didn't mention was that I'd found Mary alone in the living room the day before, listening to a Bon Iver album, clutching a throw pillow to her chest, her face wet with tears.

In the days and weeks after my diagnosis, Mary and I had clung to one another like the sole survivors of a shipwreck. Aside from our families, very few people knew about my diagnosis. Telling people hadn't been easy. A cancer diagnosis was a rarified event in our circle of friends. Life-threatening illnesses were not a part of their vernacular. They were writing books, raising children, and renovating their kitchens. Maybe they'd had a parent or grandparent succumb to the disease, but their view was from the balcony, not the front row.

And even if we'd had the words, we didn't know how to share them. In an age of Facebook and Twitter, people's lives were filtered through pics, posts, and tweets. Social media's one-dimensional note (happy!) was as forced as the smile on the face of Sharon, the nurse navigator at the first surgeon's office.

After my conversation with Patricia, I knocked on the door of Mary's office and told her of the suggestion that we gather our tribe. She took umbrage with the cultural misappropriation of the word *tribe* (of course) but leapt at the idea of a party.

Later that day, she coined the event Boobapalooza. Knowing my love of dark humor, she sent out an evite that read:

We are planning to give Catherine's boobs a little send off with some snacks and light-hearted fun, including: dark humor, boob soliloquies, breast toasts, and your favorite boob story.

The next day Mary walked down the street to the Garden of Eden, Bloomington's adult boutique, a supplier of party favors for every bachelor and bachelorette party in town. An hour later she was back home with a paper grocery bag. She sat me down at the yellow Formica table and pulled out: boob-shaped candles, boob lollipops, and balloons that inflated into a buxom twosome. Saving the best for last, she drew out a pair of pink, plastic wind-up boobs with red, mouse-sized feet. She spun the tiny black dial and giggled as the two-inch-tall bosom marched toward me across the table with a clickity-clack.

That Sunday, the day before surgery, we swung open our front door to ten of our closest friends. In came smiles, laughter, and exuberance. In each person's arms was a contribution for brunch. Cartons of orange juice, bottles of Prosecco, an egg and cheese casserole, and white cupcakes with pink frosting, each one topped with a single pink gumdrop.

My stomach lurched at the thought of all of these people coming to see me, to lend their support. I hated being the center of a group's attention. When all eyes were on me I melted into a puddle of self-consciousness—words vanished, blood rushed to my face. Mary had learned not to throw me birthday parties or call attention to me in a crowd.

But that Sunday afternoon everyone who came knew me, and no one put me on the spot. Mary mingled and greeted friends at the door while I made vats of coffee in the back corner of the kitchen. My sister, Ginny, drove up from Louisville to be a part of my support team. One by one, each of my friends worked their way back to the corner of the kitchen to say hello. Concern burned behind their eyes, but they let me drive the conversation. We talked about their gardens, their partners, and their teaching load. They asked broad questions about my health and accepted my vague answers along with a mug of French roast.

An hour later, when everyone's bellies were full of casserole and boob cupcakes, we gathered in the living room. One by one each friend spoke, told us what they hoped for us, how they'd support us, and what they, too, knew about loss, illness, and grief. The mood of friendship settled and condensed in the room, like a compote to be stored and dipped into one teaspoon at a time to sweeten the taste of what was to come.

Later that night, I took a bath. I filled the claw-foot tub, dribbled the oil, adjusted the temperature, and lowered my body into the steaming water. From the living room, I heard the faint dialogue of an old *Star Trek* episode, Mary's anti-anxiety medication. I reached for a washcloth, drug it across the surface of the steaming water, and lay it to rest over my breasts. The weight of the water-soaked cloth was reassuring. The scent of lemongrass filled the room. The candlelight reflected off the droplets of bath oil floating on the water's surface.

I took stock of the body stretched out before me. My dad's wide feet. My mom's muscular legs. My short waist. My breasts floated ever so slightly in the bathwater, half submerged under the white washcloth. I didn't know how to say goodbye.

Was I making a mistake?

Was this too radical of a choice?

Would I regret losing them both when I could have saved one?

There was no right answer. I lay in the bath until the water was tepid, until the pads on my fingers and toes were wrinkled and water-logged. After what seemed like forever I yanked the plug out of the rusted drain and wrung the washcloth dry as the gulping sound of pipes sucking water filled the room.

CHAPTER 11

In the turbulent days after my diagnosis, repeating the same dismal news to well-meaning friends and family members had become unbearable, so I started a blog. Besides, it was 2009. Blogging was the platform du jour. The blog was meant to be a central location for posting logistics, like test results and surgery dates, but it quickly grew into a confessional. Writing allowed me to tap into a voice that I otherwise struggled to find. Call it an occupational hazard but sharing my thoughts from the safety of my keyboard was easier than talking face-to-face with friends and family. Equal parts bravado and cowardice.

The blog would become a source of tension between me and Mary. Not because things I wrote were too personal or too revealing but because I didn't know how to tell her what I was thinking until it popped out in a blog post. My innermost fears about my cancer and the upcoming surgery found their way to my fingers long before they reached my lips. I'd write a new blog post and push the "publish" button from the bedroom, and she'd see a notification pop up on her laptop in the adjoining room. She'd read the innermost workings of my mind along with the rest of my blog's subscribers. Later, she'd tell me how hurt she was, but, at the time, I struggled to share my thoughts with her in real time. My cancer diagnosis had been a one-way ticket to the planet of the infirm, and she was root bound in the planet of the healthy. She wanted a guest pass to my planet, and I didn't know how to give her one.

The blog seemed a good place to post a goodbye letter to my breasts.

Dear Girls,

I feel like I hardly know you. Sure, we've been together a long time, but, like a lot of long-term couples, our relationship has evolved, deepened, and matured over time. In those early days of teenage angst, when we were first introduced, I hope you didn't pick up on my disappointment. No, it wasn't anything you did, per se. It was just, well, honestly, you were a little smaller than I'd anticipated.

While the other seventh-grade girls celebrated their new breasts with elaborate fittings at Nordstrom's, my mother marched me unceremoniously into JCPenny and handed me a bra in a box. My friends came back to school in a happy whirl of lace and underwire. I was still assembling the box's contents—a tumble of rubber bands and cotton triangles.

Okay, maybe that was a rough patch, but you and I soon settled into an easy camaraderie. Of course, no one saw much of you during the '80s, including myself. I was too busy trying to dress like Jennifer Beals. But, under all those yards of material, I knew you were there. So did the boyfriends and, later, the girlfriends. Yep, you've seen it all. You stood by while I figured out my orientation, then waited patiently as I thumbed my nose at my childbearing years, even though it meant you'd never get to nurse a baby.

I only started appreciating you when I hit my mid-30s. Something shifted and I rediscovered these cool things I had called breasts. I splurged on form-fitting shirts and sweaters. And, with Mary's encouragement, even bought a semi-sexy, halter-style yoga top last summer. When I wore that top for the first time, I noticed your graceful curves and how perfectly you met my desire for understated femininity. For the first time in my life, I took joy in you. Being in my body felt akin to driving a late-model car and suddenly discovering it had a sunroof. Overnight, that one small spark of newness infused every ride with a little oomph. I'm sad to lose you.

Love,
Catherine

On the morning of the surgery we drove to Indianapolis. I don't remember the light, the noise, the NPR news headlines. I don't remember if Mary adjusted every knob on the dashboard. I had checked out of my body, ridden the elevator to the ground floor and fled. At the hospital Mary steered my abandoned shell through the front entrance, into registration, and then onto an elevator that took us to the basement.

When we stepped off, it was nearly into my mother's lap. She'd driven up from Louisville the day before and spent the night at a hotel near the hospital so she could be there at dawn. I'd asked her to come because, even though she wasn't one to show a lot of emotion, I found her presence deeply comforting. And I'd asked my father to stay behind. He'd protested, but I insisted. Some people draw comfort and energy from family rushing to the bedside, but that was not my style. I needed this surgery to be over with as little fanfare as possible. That morning, my mother got to the hospital the way she gets everywhere—thirty minutes early. So, by the time we rode the elevator down and the DING signaled the door sliding open, my mother looked as if she'd been up for hours.

Settled into a chair near the elevator, she wore forest green wool slacks, a mock turtleneck, and a navy knit cardigan. Her short curls were soft and springy—bimonthly permanents were her single concession to vanity. Propped on her nose were her coaster-sized progressives. Open on her lap was a history of WWII, historical and political nonfiction being her genre of choice. The woman was never without a book.

She knew more about world history than anyone I knew. At times like this I imagined the books both passed the time and created a bubble that kept the real world at bay. In my family, books were shields to both deflect and protect.

She stood up and smiled, as if meeting us at a favorite restaurant. I wanted my mother to wrap her arms around me and tell me that she loved me, but I got a sideways squeeze and a pat on the arm. I reminded myself how much I loved her unbreakable strength in times of crisis, as well as her kindness and deep sense of calm. She'd showed up that morning with everything she had to give, just as she always did. A few minutes later, when the nurse called my name, Mary and I stood up to leave the waiting room, and as we followed the nurse toward the pre-op area through the swinging doors, I glanced back and saw tears glistening in my mother's eyes.

After the surgery, I woke in a dim room lit by the orange, green, and red lights of medical machinery. The rhythmic beeps and buzz of monitors keeping time. A warm weight filled my palm. I turned my head to see Mary sleeping next to my bed in the room's blue-gray recliner. She was half-sitting up, curled around a pillow the nurse must have brought for her. One of her arms was threaded through the bed's metal railing, her hand holding mine, a tether should I try to float away in the night.

By morning, I woke up to the recliner back in its rightful corner and the windows streaked with rain. From the corner, my mother looked up from her book and Mary appeared in the doorway, her eyes bloodshot, her hands clasped around a Styrofoam coffee cup as if in prayer. She and my mother took turns relaying details from the prior day.

Number of lymph nodes removed: six.

Length of surgery: two hours.

Number of lymph nodes that tested positive for cancer: zero.

I made her repeat the number, my mother too, just to make sure I'd heard correctly.

"Zero," said Mary, picking up my hand from the blanket and giving it a squeeze.

Relief rinsed through my aching chest.

My cancer was thought to be early stage, but one can't know for sure until nearby lymph nodes are examined. Solid cancers spread through the lymph nodes, nodules of tissue that filter the body's waste. During the surgery, Dr. B injected a blue dye near the tumor. The first lymph node to turn blue was considered the sentinel node, meaning it was first in line to receive whatever waste products the tumor cast off. If the cancer had spread, the sentinel node would test positive. Mine was negative. Dr. B had removed the sentinel node and five others just to be safe. All tested negative for cancer, which meant my disease hadn't spread into the nodes.

A few minutes later, Dr. B strode into the room wearing a Leprechaun-green bow tie and trailing a scent of soap and hand sanitizer. He nodded at Mary and shook my mother's hand. He looked at me and reaffirmed the good news—"No positive nodes!"—then stepped to the side of the bed and, with a quick motion, lowered the metal rail.

"Let's take a look, shall we?"

He leaned over the bed. My mother slipped out into the hall. Mary stood at the end of the bed, her hand resting on the top of the blanket-mount of my foot. I was woozy. Things were moving too fast. I needed to hit the pause button, a moment to steady myself. But, ready or not, my gown was open. Dr. B touched the flesh around the incision lightly, as if seeing if the paint were dry on his latest canvas. He nodded and tsk-ed in the affirmative. I looked down.

In hindsight, maybe I'd hoped to see a snowy white field of medical-grade gauze held in place by yards of stretchy tape. But I was mistaken.

My breasts were gone. My skin was bare. No gauze. No Ace bandage. No stitches. Just two scars, neat and pink. A clear gluelike gel held the seam of my incision together. At the outside corner of each seam emerged a plastic tube. Follow the tube to its end, and you'd see a clear, plastic drain shaped like a hand-grenade.

Years later, when I recounted the unveiling to another doctor, she sucked in her breath and murmured something about how you'd never do that to someone who'd had an amputation. When I asked her what she meant, she said, "What you had was an amputation. No doctor would ever amputate someone's leg and then whip off the covering to reveal the stump. There is an entire catalog of literature about how to prepare the patient for that moment."

But that morning at the Simon Cancer Center, there was no preparation. My torso was a moonscape of loss, a no man's land of bumps and craters. My upper ribs in high relief. The structural elements of my body laid bare, a sofa with busted-out springs.

What did I think this was going to look like?

Maybe that by some miracle my chest would be smooth and flat?

That the mastectomy photos I'd seen online were all anomalies?

That I would be an exception?

And then I saw it. That damn mole. That lentil-shaped spot. The signpost I'd used to direct doctors to the lump sat undisturbed on the devastation of my chest like a cockroach that had survived a bomb blast.

"What's the matter?" asked Dr. B.

"I thought it would be gone."

"What?"

"That mole," I said, embarrassed that I thought the skin covering my breast was part of the deal, that I'd pictured mastectomy as akin to mountaintop removal, the whole mound severed from its base. Now I know that's not how the surgery worked. Dr. B had made the incisions, lifted up the skin, removed the bulk of breast tissue, laid the skin back down, trimmed the edges, and closed the wound. I had to replace my image of strip-mined mountains with one of pillowcases, able to be stuffed or unstuffed. And mine were decidedly unstuffed.

Without the buffer of breasts, my chest was as scrawny as a baby bird's. My heart, stripped of its protection, threatened to flop out of my chest, like a fish on the bottom of a boat. A part of me wondered if this was real. Maybe I was at home in our bedroom with its sage-colored walls, the dog curled in the corner, all four paws twitching as she chased rabbits.

But the plastic mattress pad was slippery and crinkly beneath my hips. The cool liquid from the IV dripped through the hot needle taped to the back of my hand. My foot felt the steady pressure of Mary's palm, my eyes traveled up the length of her arm and met her gaze. She smiled a low-voltage version of a crooked smile. Behind her bookish glasses, her red-rimmed eyes told me she, too, was relieved that my breast cancer scare was almost over. For the second time that day, she tethered me to the earth, anchored me when I wanted to float into the haze of panic and uncertainty.

Two hours later, a nurse pushed a towering metal cart into my hospital room. "Mastectomy?" she called out, as if she were taking roll and mastectomy was my new name. Mary and I exchanged looks from across the room. Mom lifted her eyes from the pages of her book.

The cart, piled high with plastic-wrapped bundles, stopped beside my bed. The nurse popped out from behind it. She was my mother's age, her hair arranged in similar curls that were more salt than pepper. Pinned to the top of her head was an old-fashioned nurse's hat, a vision in starched geometry. She eyeballed me, rifled through the plastic bags, and pulled something from the bottom of the pile.

With both hands, she dug her fingers into the belly of the bag and tore it open the way you might break open a party-size bag of chips. Inside was a post-mastectomy camisole. She sidled up to the bedside. The metal railing fell with a clang. With the experience of someone who'd done this thousands of times, she slipped the hospital gown up and off of me. Then she scrunched the camisole's fabric up, from bottom to top, popped it over my head, and wiggled it down over my body, a mother putting a sock on a toddler.

As she tugged the soft fabric over my torso, my nervous system quieted. Only then did I notice how I'd been bracing myself against the world. That the nerve endings in my skin were stripped and exposed, like the stump of a tooth prepped for a crown. The muscles of my jaw, neck, and shoulders softened. The camisole had two pockets to hold the drains—a place to tuck the awkward bulbs so as not to get tangled up in sheets or clothes. My mother nodded approvingly. Mary smiled. I thanked the nurse. She told me there was more to come.

She reached deep into the bottom of her cart and returned to my bedside with two cottony white footballs. She tugged open the neckline of my camisole and began to stuff one of the footballs into place. As she pushed and pulled, my arms braced against the bed.

"Um, wait," I said. "I don't . . . really."

"What?" she said.

"I don't really . . ."

She drew back, parked her hands on her wide hips. "Most ladies won't leave the hospital without their breast forms," she said.

"No really, I'm fine," I said.

The fireplug of a nurse swung around to look at my mother to get her thoughts on the situation. My mother stuck a finger in her book and flapped a hand loosely at the footballs. "Don't bother with that, she doesn't need those."

"Well, I'll just leave 'em here at the foot of the bed, and you can take 'em on home," said the nurse. "You paid for 'em so you might as well keep 'em." She placed the two footballs next to my feet before circling back to the front of her cart. I got the feeling she wasn't the kind of woman who liked leaving a job half done, but she seemed to know she was outnumbered and left the room.

When we could no longer hear the rattling of the cart and the squeak of her shoes in the hall, we all exhaled. I want to say the three of us shared a much-needed laugh, that my mom squinted her eyes and leaned her head back, covering her open-mouthed giggle with her hand. I want to say that Mary let out one of her spirited "ho-HOs," the sound of delight and surprise she often made before doubling over in laughter, but instead my memory is clouded by the strangeness of the moment. Staring at the breast forms at the foot of the bed, I couldn't stop thinking about how they were three times bigger than the peach-sized breasts I'd sacrificed the day before. How the mastectomy nurse, like the breast surgeons, hadn't paused to ask me how I wanted to present my body to the world, but moved on autopilot to return their definition of femininity to my now gender-ambiguous chest.

A week later, I read Audre Lorde's account of her mastectomy in 1978. On the day after her mastectomy, Lorde, a poet and breast cancer activist, was visited by a "kindly woman" who offered her "a very upbeat message and a little prepared packet containing . . . a wad of lamb's wool pressed into a pale-pink breast-shaped pad." Of the scene, she wrote: "Breast prostheses are offered to women after surgery in much the same way that candy is offered to babies after an injection." I was struck by how little had changed in thirty years. How little space women were given for mourning. How strong the medical community's insistence was that a woman's body conform.

CHAPTER 12

On that first night home from the hospital, back inside the white rectangle of a house, sitting at the yellow table and staring at the leafless maple tree in the front yard, I ate the home-cooked meal Mary put in front of me—thick lentil soup, a green salad, and double-chocolate brownies. This was remarkable namely because Mary didn't cook. But she had generous and empathetic colleagues who coordinated to cook and deliver dinner to us over the next couple of weeks. That night I was overcome with relief and gratitude that someone had spent an afternoon preparing a meal for us. More food arrived with every passing day. Deep-dish casseroles and creamy quiches with flaky crusts. Delicate vegetable broths and hearty winter stews. Eggplant Parmesan with crusty garlic bread. Every dish steeped in love and caring. So why did I begin to dread the drop-off?

The doorbell's late-afternoon DING DONG sent Emma on a barking jag, her toenails digging into the hardwood floors as she ripped through the house. Mary would leap from her chair and race after the dog. The door swung open to a cheerful friend who bustled into our small, cold kitchen. Bubbling over with energy, vitality, and news from the University, the friend would splay open her canvas grocery bag and withdraw a small feast. Out came a Dutch oven fragrant with minestrone soup, a salad made with the spring greens she'd picked from her greenhouse, a fruit smoothie for dessert or even breakfast the next morning. Instructions were given on how to reheat the main dish. And then we'd all shuffle into the living room and sit on the brown couch to exchange quips of news and gossip. I grew to loathe these visits and, in turn, myself for being so bitchy and ungrateful. But the contrast between my friends' lives and mine was too much to bear. Healthy and vibrant, they burst on the scene with energy to spare. During sofa chats they shared stories of stubborn children, recalcitrant dogs, moles burrowing into vegetable patches. I'd smile, nod, wrap my hands around my mug of tea, lift it to my lips. My marionette body nodding at the appropriate times, piping up with the occasional "really?" or "wow!" while my cancer-patient self peered at the scene through the distancing binoculars of illness.

Sitting between me and the visitor, Mary did her best to carry the conversation, her hand squeezing my thigh when she noticed I'd floated beyond earshot. But even Mary's Olympian patience grew thin, and sometimes, after the person left, she'd snap at me about my inability to focus or my stinginess at not having offered the guest even a crumb of conversation. Then she'd stomp upstairs to her office and I'd slouch, dazed, on the edge of the couch, holding a mug of cold tea, confused about how I'd lost traction on my life. The surgery had gone well. I was only stage 1. I should have been thankful, relieved. But I was grieving my breasts and my old self.

Before now, I'd been on the giving end of these sickbed visits. I liked being the one who dropped off the hot meal, who basked in the warm feelings of one's generosity. I'm embarrassed to say that more than once, upon making my exit, I'd felt a small shudder of gratitude for the healthy body I often took for granted.

For the days following the surgery, my mother stayed in Bloomington to help, spending days at the house and nights at a nearby hotel to give us space. On the fourth day she suggested we walk Emma to the park. She didn't care for dogs, so she must have been bored silly. This was a woman who rarely sat down, who could garden from dawn to dusk, who had dessert made and the first steps of dinner completed by 9 a.m. For four days she'd been parked on the brown couch. I noticed she'd finished her book on WWII and consumed every lick of reading material on our sparse coffee table, including *Anticancer: A New Way of Life*. The book was a heartfelt gift from one of my editors that I couldn't bring myself to open. If I already had cancer, wouldn't it only make me sad to read about how I might have prevented it in the first place?

"Sure, let's walk to the park." I said, taking Emma's leash from its hook on the wall. The dog scrambled off her bed, her nails tapping on the wood floor like typewriter keys.

"I'll steer," announced my mother, who'd never walked a dog in her life. I wasn't supposed to strain my arms, so I reluctantly handed the leash to my mother and glowered at Emma to behave herself. I'd never imagined my mother walking my dog. But I hadn't imagined a lot of things.

Outside, the air spoke of rain. We walked in silence toward the park, our steps measured by the soft jangle of dog tags. My chest was numb. This was my first time out in public since the surgery. I crossed my arms. Cradled my fresh wounds like a baby. I prayed no one I knew would see us. I had no energy or words for small talk.

The Honda CRV crept up from behind, its engine eerily quiet.

"Hey! You're up! Looking good," called Lorraine. She leaned over to look at me through the passenger-side window. My mouth forced itself into a smile-like shape. The dog whined and strained toward the car while my mother's arthritic hands clamped onto the leash. I hadn't had time to tell my mother about Lorraine or explain that she was my neighbor and the only woman I knew who'd dealt with her breast cancer by having a double mastectomy without reconstruction. And that, since her surgery the year before, Lorraine liked to brag about how she had the perfect pair of breasts. Perfect because they were in her sock drawer, ready to be pulled out and worn on special occasions the way other women might wear pearls or lipstick.

Before I could say any of this, Lorraine tossed her head back and let out a raucous laugh. "You're one of us now. We flat-chested chicks gotta stick together!"

And with that she pulled away, the pink-ribbon decal on her bumper glinting in the sun. In that moment, I desperately wanted to be Lorraine. I wanted to be happy-go-lucky. I wanted to be the good breast cancer patient. The chin-up, move-on, get-over-it type. I wanted to throw back my head, joke about my flat chest, and order a pair of special-occasion tits and bed them down in my sock drawer. But that wasn't me. Not only was I not like Lorraine, I wasn't like any breast cancer patient I'd met either in person or online. I wasn't focused on reconstruction like the other young women in the breast cancer forums. I wasn't my mother's best friend, Bonnie, content to pass as having a body untouched by cancer. I certainly wasn't even close to Kris Carr's crazy, sexy persona.

Why couldn't I just join a team?

The initial days after the surgery were spent trying not to tangle myself in the plastic drainage tubes that sprouted from either side of my chest. Each tube ended in a hollow bulb, the size of a Meyer lemon, that collected runoff from the incision site. The tubes were sutured in place, and the slightest pressure, in the form of a pull or a tug, sent a red-hot poker of pain into my ribs.

Most of the time the tubes were coiled and stuffed into the shallow pockets of my hospital-issued camisole. I looked like a kangaroo with two joeys. But when the extra feet of tubing sprung from my pockets, a loose loop would often catch on a drawer pull as I walked from the kitchen to the dining room table or the tubing would get caught on the top button of my jeans when I pulled them down to use the bathroom. And BAM! A sharp jolt on the end of the line that made me suck in my breath, freeze, and slowly reverse out of whatever I was doing. To ward off such sneak attacks, I started creeping through the house like a cat burglar.

The drains had to be emptied and cleaned. Mary, who prided herself on her lack of squeamishness about bodily fluids, volunteered for the job. Twice a day we'd meet in the downstairs bathroom. As she arranged supplies on top of the vanity, I'd sit on the lid of the toilet, next to the claw-foot tub. With a scientist's precision, she'd hold each drain up to the light, chart the amount of fluid, jot the number on a notepad, empty the drain, and apply a fresh bandage to the exit wound.

I was thirty-eight, Mary thirty-nine. Yes, we'd hoped to reach old age together, but we hadn't planned on being one another's caretaker so soon. Five years before, we'd had a commitment ceremony at the Peterson Palace and invited a hundred loved ones. On that crisp October morning, amidst golden mums and sunflower bouquets, we'd worn white, walked down the grand staircase and out into my mother's garden. We beamed at one another through our tears and promised to love and care for one another.

Back in the bathroom, my squirming made Mary nervous. Afraid of hurting me, her fingers fumbled. She yanked on the tube, pulling it straight out and away from my body, causing the sutures to strain their grip.

"Ow! Jesus, just give it to me. I'll do it myself!"

She opened her mouth to protest. Then she handed me the drain and walked out.

In the days that followed, Mary's protective side flared. I wasn't to lift more than ten pounds until my drains were removed, which meant no yoga poses that put weight on my arms, no dog walking, and no grocery shopping. Her request that I not go to the grocery alone was the hardest rule to accept. I loved shopping for food almost as much as I loved eating it. Every trip to the store was an adventure in possibility. Every item held the promise of a delicious meal in the waiting. I knew every aisle of Bloomingfoods co-op by heart. I noticed when they added a new variety of rice to the bulk bin section or put a new curry paste on the shelf. I followed the change of seasons as reflected in the produce, running my hands over pyramids of ripe peaches, nectarines, and avocados, pressing my fingertips into each fruit to search for the elasticity that signaled perfect ripeness.

After much arguing and exasperated sighs, she agreed to let me go but only if I promised to follow specific protocol. First, I must use a cart *not* a hand-held basket. Second, at checkout, I must ask a bagger to walk me to my car. Third, at the car, the bagger must lift the bags from the cart into the trunk. Finally, when I returned home, the groceries had to stay in the car until Mary fetched them for me. This final step was the most fraught.

Autonomy was the WD-40 that oiled the wheels of our relationship. We were willing to do anything for the other but only in our own sweet time (emergencies notwithstanding). Because Mary was often working when I got home, she'd register my request then shoo me away from her office door saying she needed "just one more minute to finish up this email." An hour later, I'd go outside to find a soupy pint of Ben and Jerry's in the backseat of the car. As I cleaned up the mess, I reminded myself that it was only for a couple of weeks before things would be back to normal.

One week after my double mastectomy, my mom was back in Louisville, Mary was back on campus, and I was embracing convalescence on the brown couch. That's how I came to be watching an Oprah show on medical errors. Dr. Oz was the guest.

Bear with me. This was early in his career as a TV persona, and he hadn't endorsed any cuckoo products or made any one of a number of questionable remarks. He was still a very credible cardiologist. We'd spoken multiple times for articles I'd written about heart disease. He was humble and generous with an uncanny ability to put complex medical information in terms that were easy to understand. In our interviews, he was never cocky or rushed but instead down-to-earth and patient.

So, with an empty afternoon stretched in front of me, and a yen for medical tough-luck stories, I turned up the volume and settled in for an hourlong show on medical errors. Oprah had on a guest named Molly who had had a mastectomy after a breast cancer diagnosis. Eight days after her surgery, Molly learned there had been a mistake at the lab. Slides from her biopsy were switched with another patient's. That patient had breast cancer, not Molly. Molly's biopsy had been benign. The mastectomy had been unnecessary.

I shifted on the couch. The drains tugged at the incisions on my chest. Emma lifted her head, looked out the window, and growled.

Jesus, could that have happened to me?

Running back through my ordeal, I knew I'd been meticulous in finding the doctor with the best credentials. I remembered how Dr. B had sent my biopsy to the hospital's lab, a safety measure to double-check the initial report from St. Vincent's. How he'd strode into my hospital room in his bright green bow tie and assured me and Mary that my surgery had been a success. How he'd reported that the half-dozen lymph nodes he'd removed were cancer-free. My surgery had gone as well as I could have hoped. Right?

As the show went on, more guests shared horrific stories of medical errors. At the end of the hour, Dr. Oz looked straight into the camera and implored viewers to speak up if they found themselves on the receiving side of a doctor's error. It was as if he was looking right at me when he said, "Remember, you are the world's foremost expert on your body. Trust what it's telling you." Then the camera panned back to Molly who was hugging Oprah. And, as I hit the power-off button on the remote, I offered up a silent prayer of thanks that my surgery had gone well.

CHAPTER 13

The next day, Dr. B burst into the exam room like a radiator on the cusp of overheating. It was one week after my double mastectomy, and Mary and I had returned to the Simon Cancer Center to get my drains removed and to hear the full pathology report.

In the days since my surgery I'd tried not to think too much about the amputation of my breasts—how my breast tissue might have jiggled on the stainless-steel tray, how my breasts might have been bagged, labeled, and transported to the hospital's pathology lab. In some dreams my amputated breasts looked like beached jellyfish lying lifeless in the sun. In other dreams the pathologist strained my breast tissue through a sieve like a California Gold Rush miner panning dirt in search of precious nuggets.

Today Dr. B stood in front of me, waving the pages of the pathology report like a victory flag. "Good news!"

Cathy edged into the room and took her customary stance by the door as Dr. B laid out the findings. He chose words like *minuscule* and *tiny* to describe the nuggets of cancer found at the bottom of the pathologist's sieve.

Minuscule?

Tiny?

My stomach quivered. These words were not mine. They did not describe my tumor, the shard of glass lodged under my skin. A grain of sand is tiny. A speck of dust is minuscule. My lump had been neither tiny nor miniscule. The surgeon felt it. I felt it. Mary felt it. Even Beth felt it. Those adjectives never came to mind.

But it was clear in his tone and body language that none of that mattered now. All of our previous knowledge and my body's knowing had been usurped by a new, all-knowing truth—the truth of the pathology report. The report was indisputable. Black and white, full of scientific measurements, signed off on by multiple white coats. People who supposedly knew better. The patient's place was not to question the pathology report.

"You don't understand," said Dr. B when he saw my confusion. "This is the best possible scenario."

I wanted nothing more than to meet Dr. B in the land of excitement. To look at the report and give it more weight than my sixth sense, but I couldn't do it. My footing felt wobbly, my stomach woozy. A crack in the earth—dark and ominous—was opening beneath me.

"But . . . the lump," I stammered.

From her seat against the wall, Mary said something to Dr. B. At least I think she did. Her lips moved but her words were muffled by the rush of blood in my ears.

Dr. B waved the report at us like a get-out-of-jail-free card. "It says right here the cancer was negligible," he said. "Don't you understand? This is the best outcome you could hope for."

I swallowed my questions as he and Cathy prepped the instrument tray.

He was telling me I'd won the cancer jackpot. Why was I questioning my luck?

No one had explained to me how my drains, these skinny hoses snaking from my sides, would be extracted from my body, and, per my ostrichlike approach to this ordeal, I'd been hesitant to ask.

Dr. B held the surgical scissors. The metal blade pressed against my skin. Snip. The black suture fastening the tube to my skin was gone. He stood up, placed one palm flat against my ribs, and took a firm hold on the tube with the other hand. And, with the practiced skill of a fisherman gutting a fish, pulled firm and fast (the word *yank* comes to mind, but it was more precise than a yank). I picture it now as if watching someone pull the cord on a lawnmower, knowing exactly what angle and how much pressure to apply to the cord to get the job done. The tube exited through the hole in my left side. And then it was done.

"One down, one to go," he said.

Again. Snip. Steady. Pull. Fffsshhhtt . . . the plastic tube whipped through my body. A burn traced through me, like the lit fuse of a firecracker. With a flick of his wrist, Dr. B aimed the tube at a nearby trashcan and let go. Two points.

Then he peeled off his Latex gloves. Cathy cleared the instruments from the tray. The mood in the room was one of satisfaction. I sat up. Without the drains, my chest was light and empty. Reflexively, I ran my fingertips across the spot where the lump had been. I wanted assurance that the cancer was gone, that I could move on with my life. Muscle memory propelled my fingers to the place where they'd wheedled cancer like a worry bead, near the small mole, the lump's trusty sentinel. Then my fingertips brushed the skin. Stopped. They caught on something. A shard of glass. A broken tooth.

Dr. B tapped the bottom of my file on the countertop to neaten the edges of the papers inside. The gesture was one of finality. His work here was done. Another woman was tumor-free. A satisfied customer.

My fingertips were magnetized to the bump on the left side of my chest. I clambered for my voice.

"A lump. There's still a lump."

Mary's eyes leapt up from her notebook.

Dr. B paused, my folder in his hands, his mind on his next patient no doubt. "I'm sure it's nothing," he said, waving away my concern with a shake of his head as he moved toward the door. "I'll see you back in two weeks to check on the incisions."

My mouth went dry. A thin coat of sweat sprung up beneath my arms. Panic rose in my chest. I fought the urge to grab his sleeve. He couldn't leave. Not now. Not with the lump still inside me.

"I need you to feel it," I said.

The sour look on Dr. B's face told me my "lump talk" was putting a damper on his morning. He'd performed a textbook double mastectomy. The patient was healing. He was only moments away from handing her off to an oncologist. But somewhere in the last few minutes, she'd somersaulted from happy customer to hypochondriac. I could almost see the dismissal in his eyes. He opened his mouth as if to say something, then closed it. He glanced at Mary in the corner, who had put her notebook down. She was spring loaded for a fight. He sighed, put the folder down, and took a step toward me. He placed the blunt tips of his fingers on my chest. A flash of curiosity crossed his face, then vanished.

"I'm sure it's nothing," he shrugged. "Probably just fatty tissue."

He turned and reached for the door, a gesture indicating closure.

"Fatty tissue?" I croaked in disbelief.

Cathy shifted uneasily. Maybe she was eager for closure, too. Weren't we all? But I'd found my voice, and I wasn't letting either one of them out of my sight.

"I'm not leaving with this lump." My panic was morphing into white, hot anger.

Dr. B looked at his watch then back at me.

"If it would make you happy, we could biopsy it."

Happy? If it would make me happy?

The thought of a biopsy did not make me happy at all. A biopsy meant offering up my aching chest to the CLACK of the pellet gun. It meant wearing the cancer broach home and waiting. Results would take days. Besides, the point of a goddamn biopsy was to find out if a lump was cancerous. I knew the answer to this question.

But it's the same fucking lump! I wanted to scream.

Mary's voice sluiced the air. "Can she get another mammogram? The lump had a metal tag. If it's the same lump, the tag will show up."

Dr. B let out a long, slow breath. "Fine."

Cathy picked up the phone mounted on the wall of the exam room, called the hospital's mammography center, and told them the situation. She hung up and looked at me and Mary. The schedule was tight, but if I could get down there right away they could fit me in.

Getting from the cancer center to the radiology department was like threading your way through one of the mind-boggling corn mazes that popped up around Bloomington every autumn. The two buildings, the century-old Indiana University Hospital, and the brand new Simon Cancer Center, were connected but at odd angles and with rough seams of battleship-gray double doors, mismatched flooring, and endless hallways steeped in the rancid smell of the cafeteria's deep fryer.

Mary and I raced from one building to the next, stopping only long enough to confer with nods and jerks of the head about whether to go left or right, take the elevator up or down. After what felt like a mile-long sprint, the mammography center came into view. We threw ourselves at the receptionist's desk as if across a track-and-field finish line.

She looked up, popping her gum. "Do you have a copy of your previous mammogram?"

Mary and I spun toward one other.

This exact scenario—records in multiple places—was something I'd hoped to avoid by picking a hospital with everything under one roof.

"You don't have access to that information?" I asked.

"Nope," she said. "Different system."

Mary stopped pawing through her backpack. She didn't have it with her.

"Cathy has it. I'll be right back," she said to me as she sprinted away.

Now I was alone.

A nurse called me back into the patient locker room. My robot arms took off my street clothes, hung them in a locker, and put on a hospital gown. A few minutes later I faced a mammography machine for only the second time in my life. But this time I had no breasts.

How was this going to work?

The technician arrived. She introduced herself and began to prep the machine, adjusting the flat, glass paddles. When she indicated she was ready for me, I stepped forward and untied the gown. Looking at my fresh scars, my concave chest, the nurse pursed her lips and let out a low whistle.

"So, why?"

I told her about the double mastectomy, the fatty tissue, and the metal tag inserted at St. Vincent's six weeks earlier.

Her fingertips touched the lump. The confusion melted off her face. A lump was something she could work with.

She told me to wrap my arms around the machine's vertical steel body. Then she used the weight of her body to press against my back. Together we shoved, squeezed, and pressed a small pad of flesh between the machine's dinner-plate-sized paddles. My chest was still numb from the surgery, so I jammed it against the machine hard enough to crack a rib.

But I didn't care.

The truth was inside that tiny pad of tissue. Goddamn it, I was not leaving until I could prove my body was right, that it was the same lump, that the cancer was still inside of me.

"I think you're in," she said, as she eased away. "Don't move. Don't even breathe."

The machine whirred. Lights blinked.

"Okay. We got it," she said. The paddles relaxed their grip on my body.

A few minutes later, a radiologist entered the room. This was not standard procedure. Radiologists and patients didn't stand shoulder to shoulder waiting for the results of a mammogram. But nothing about this situation was standard. The air inside the windowless room grew taut as we stared at the black monitor. "As soon as the image is processed, this is where it will appear," she said tapping the frame. She was trim and fit, her brown hair held back in a loose twist. She exuded a calm perfectionism. I gathered the thin hospital gown around myself even tighter, less for warmth and more for protection against what I knew was coming.

Ordinarily, I wouldn't presume to know a cancerous lump if I saw one. But that day I knew exactly what I was looking for. The monitor began to flicker. Together the radiologist and I leaned forward and held our breath. Then the black-and-white image of my mammogram leapt onto the screen.

The metal tag blazed center screen. I could almost hear the CLACK, the UFO hovering over the rolling landscape of my soft tissue. The radiologist crossed her arms and squinted at the screen. "Who was your surgeon again?" she asked. I answered. She shook her head. Dr. B was the director of breast cancer surgical oncology at the most reputable cancer center in the state. He'd done hundreds of mastectomies. Mine was not a difficult case. This was a brazen error.

A red-hot cauldron of rage bubbled inside me. The radiologist deposited me in an empty exam room to wait while she made her report. The room was long and narrow, a shoebox in a land of cubes. The radiology department was on the basement level but this room had high windows along the far wall. The view was of a pebble-lined drainage area between two buildings. The weight of the hospital pressed down from above. Among the smooth rocks, a lone pigeon pecked for food. Above, a slice of dark-gray sky ran between the buildings.

Where was Mary? What was taking her so long?

Adrenaline snapped and crackled in my veins. Unable to stop, think, or sit still, I lurched from one end of the room to the next, my hands balled into fists, my body trembling. Among the cascade of thoughts tumbling through my head was the memory of Molly, from the Oprah Show, and Dr. Oz's words about medical errors.

Footsteps and voices in the hall. Mary burst through the door, her face a swirl of agony. Later she would tell me that the mammography nurses didn't know where I'd gone. The radiologist had gone back to her office. No one knew she'd put me in the long room at the end of the hall and closed the door. Mary had been dashing through the halls quizzing every nurse and technician about my whereabouts for the past five minutes. She tossed the manila envelope with the mammogram, a document we no longer needed, onto the exam table and pulled me toward her. I tucked my head into the crook of her neck and wailed.

Soon we had to retrace our steps through the hospital corridors. This time my steps were leaden, my vision blurred by tears. With her arm around my shoulder, Mary led me up elevators, down hallways, and through swarms of doctors, medical students, and visitors descending on the cafeteria for lunch.

Back inside Dr. B's exam room, my body crumpled into one of the black plastic chairs along the wall. Mary sat vigil beside me.

The walls squeezed in. The lights buzzed. My arms wrapped tightly across my chest. My mind whirled from question to question like a marble bouncing around a roulette wheel.

How was this possible?

How did he remove both my breasts but miss the lump?

The pathology report found cancer, but the lump was still under my skin, so what was the cancer they found?

Was it more cancer or had he nicked the lump?

Disturbing a tumor was a grave mistake. Cutting into the capsule was like kicking a beehive. If he had nicked the tumor, millions of cancer cells could have been released into my body.

Together we waited.

Footsteps in the hall.

The door swung open.

Our eyes locked on him, his short, square body, his small eyes. The skin of his face was pasty, a sheen of sweat across his forehead. The air inside the closet-sized room thickened with the unspoken.

He marched to the wall, clamped the new mammogram film to the board, and flipped on the light.

The metal tag jumped.

"We need to get you back to surgery right away." His voice was hard.

The floor gave way beneath me, and I was looking up at him from the bottom of a well. His face was distant, removed, confused as to how I had fallen.

"Cathy? Where's Cathy?" he barked.

She stepped into the doorway.

"Let's get another surgery lined up."

He yanked the film off the wall. Mary tightened her grip on my hand. I'd handed him my body. Trusted him with my life. He'd not only flubbed the surgery but was now refusing to acknowledge his mistake.

"How does something like this even happen?" I whispered.

He swiveled to face us head-on—Mary and I sitting in a heap against the wall.

His jaw was clenched. A thin blue vein popped across his glistening forehead. "This is highly unusual. I've never had this happen before. I'll fix it. I'll go in through the same incision. There won't be another scar."

I was a mistake he was eager to correct, not for my benefit but for his own. I wanted to remind him of his "fatty tissue" remark, about how he'd dismissed my concern with a pat on the head, but an ocean of grief washed over me. Grief for every breast cancer patient who'd ever been ignored, dismissed, or labeled as angry or anxious. Grief for every woman who'd been told she had "nothing to worry about" and sent home with cancer gnawing at her insides. Grief for the women sent to early graves by doctors who are never held accountable.

From beside me, Mary voiced the words I could not. "We need you to say you're sorry."

The prior week, shaken by Oprah's exposé on medical errors, I'd mentioned the show to Mary. Telling her about Molly's mistaken mastectomy. About the experts who'd underscored the importance of hearing doctors apologize and take ownership of mistakes.

Mary had remembered. She knew I needed him to own his error, and she wasn't going to leave until he did.

No one moved.

There we were, the three of us, stuffed into the exam room, Cathy's shadow at the door. Me drowning in disbelief. Mary laser-focused and poised on the plastic chair, her eyes boring holes into the surgeon's face.

Dr. B swallowed. He looked down, shifted the folder he was holding into his other hand. Then he looked up, his eyes brimming with tears. "I'm so sorry."

We drove the fifty miles back to Bloomington in shock, the cancerous broach in place. It was Wednesday. My new surgery date was Monday. Days of waiting, sitting with the incredulousness of what happened.

The next day, bolted to her office chair, pouring over the pathologist's report, Mary jotted down question after question. Synapses firing, seeking meaningful answers to impossible questions, this was how she coped. She put her pain to the side to deal with the crisis at hand. I was struck dumb, pinned by the weight of the surgeon's mistake and its implications, aimless in my wanderings from brown couch to white desk to yellow table. After assembling a dozen questions, Mary called Dr. B on the private number he'd given her the day before. Her voice was stern, her words clipped. My memory of the call is fuzzy, but I remember Mary's fierceness and my deep sense of her love for me.

We'll never know how Dr. B missed the lump, but here's one version of what might have happened. He sliced a single, straight line across the center of my breast and lifted up the skin to reach the breast tissue underneath. The tumor was close to the skin's surface. Perhaps the tumor came up with the top layer of skin and tissue. Perhaps he scraped out the breast tissue underneath. At some point he removed the six lymph nodes the tumor most likely drained to—the sentinel node and associates. And then, perhaps, he laid the skin back down atop my chest, smoothed it down, trimmed the excess, closed the incision, and went to the other side. Of course, this is my own speculation pieced together from his description. What is clear is that he made a mistake. He missed a step. One could say he missed *the* step. He took my breasts and left the breast cancer behind.

Here's what still haunts me: my breast cancer surgery should have been a resounding success. My lump was palpable. I'd found it early. By all measures the cancer was contained. Excellent health insurance granted me access to the best doctors in the region. I had the know-how to interview three surgeons, ask discerning questions, and choose the one with the most expertise. I'd even had input from Lance Armstrong's oncologist, the doctor who'd successfully treated the most famous cancer patient of my generation. On top of all of that, I was a women's health journalist, for god's sake. If anyone knew how to get good health care, it should have been me. If this could happen to me, what could happen to women with crappy health insurance, women who didn't have the privilege of interviewing multiple surgeons, women without a partner to lean on?

At its core, a life-threatening illness is the ultimate loss of control. The body—the one thing you are handed at birth and must look after until death—is under siege from within. I sought to regain some semblance of control by finding the best surgeon. Other breast cancer patients try to regain control by eating the perfect diet, taking the perfect combination of supplements, or reconstructing the perfect breasts. But eventually, you're reminded that control is an illusion.

Mistakes are inevitable because surgeons are human. Can you lower the odds of a mistake? Yes, by finding an experienced surgeon. As director of surgical breast oncology, Dr. B had done hundreds, if not thousands, of lumpectomies and mastectomies. But clearly experience doesn't guarantee perfection. Maybe his familiarity with the procedure had led to complacency. Or maybe he was cocky. On the morning of my surgery he'd been running late, the OR nurses making excuses as minutes ticked by. "Caught in traffic," they said. "Here any minute," they called out. When he had finally rushed through the door, he looked flushed and frazzled. Within fifteen minutes we were in surgery.

Later, he would admit he didn't pay much attention to the lump's location, assuming if he removed my breasts that the lump would be nestled inside, a pea in a mattress. During the surgery, when he sent my breast tissue to the pathologist, traces of cancer were found. He assumed those traces and the lump were one and the same and proceeded to close.

That weekend, Mary crossed the hall from her office to mine, bringing me the phone. "Your parents want to talk." She'd been keeping them updated, but I hadn't spoken to them since the mistake. I could barely make sense of what had happened for myself. How would I answer their questions? "They just need to hear your voice, honey," she said softly. "They need to know you're okay."

My father would be in the living room, with his feet up, horizontal in his recliner. My mother would be swaddled in her bathrobe, the one with the pink and yellow stripes, listening on the extension in the kitchen. This time she wouldn't be washing dishes. She'd be seated at the table, a forgotten cup of Lipton tea at her elbow. She'd poke a finger in her free ear and hold the phone to the other, her eyes closed in concentration. She, too, would want to understand.

Confusion and anger streaked their voices, even as they tried to stay calm. "We don't understand. Why go back to the same surgeon

who messed up? Why not go to the experts? Board a plane, go to a nationally renowned cancer center in Texas or Massachusetts? Why stay in Indiana?" prodded my mother.

"I know a lawyer," my father fumed, "I'll sue your surgeon's ass."

My mouth fish-gulped for answers.

I eyed Mary who'd stayed nearby, knowing I might need a quick escape from the conversation.

At some point in the past few weeks, Mary had become my fixer. Whereas I'd once been the confident health journalist, the person my family members called when they needed a quick answer to a basic health question or help researching a perplexing diagnosis, breast cancer had turned me into a fragile shell of a person who couldn't hold her own on the phone.

I made a quick excuse to my parents and held the phone out to Mary. "Please?"

She nodded, took it, and retreated back to her office speaking softly into the receiver. She had a knack for talking with my parents, especially my father. He respected her smarts and her sound judgment. Unlike me, she never snapped at his old-fashioned paternalism. In truth, she'd won him over five years earlier by taking him out to lunch and asking for my hand. That long-ago meal at Lynn's Paradise Cafe, a preface to our commitment ceremony at my parent's house the following year, had endeared Mary to my father forever. To my sisters' consternation, he liked to remind them that neither of their husbands had afforded him that antiquated courtesy. He'd been Mary's biggest booster ever since, and she had empathy and patience for him when my reserves were running low.

Needing to distance myself from their conversation, I went downstairs and began washing dishes. The warmth of the water running in the sink, the squishiness of the yellow sponge, the hit of lemon in the detergent. I sought comfort in monotony.

My parents had a point. How could I trust the same surgeon who'd

just made such a terrible mistake? But my gut told me there would be no finding someone new. All momentum for Internet research, phone calls, and arranging consultations was lost. Travel took energy, and I had none to spare. The job was botched and no one knew better what went wrong and how to fix it than the man who fucked it up in the first place.

I'm tempted to say I wanted to give him another chance, but that's not quite right. More accurately, I needed to be done with it. I needed to stop parading through surgeon's offices, explaining what happened and wondering if they'd know how to fix it. My faith in surgeons—him or anyone else—was beyond repair. I just needed it to be easy. And I needed it to be over.

On Monday we retraced our steps to the hospital in Indianapolis. Dr. B was stone-faced. No smiles, no winks, no platitudes. In the pre-op room, his hand rested on my shoulder, thick and heavy as a bookend. "I'm going to make this right," he said.

And so followed another trip to the operating room, a repeat of the first surgery—removal of more breast tissue and, finally, removal of the lump itself.

Later, friends would ask me, "So, how does one have a second mastectomy? If your breast was already gone, what did he remove?"

Removing a breast is not as simple as it sounds. The surgery is not as simple as, say, cutting out a gallbladder or an appendix. While the structures of the mammary-gland network reside in the breast, breast tissue is marbled throughout the chest and looks like any other tissue. No mastectomy can remove 100 percent of a woman's breast tissue. So, that day, Dr. B hollowed me out even more.

Later that night, back in Bloomington, my Dad sent Mary the name of a lawyer and implored her to talk some sense into me. Knowing I wanted to put the mistake behind me, Mary never showed me the email, but she did tell me about it years later.

I was not a litigious person. Retribution did not interest me. Was I pissed? Yes. Would suing him for some unspecified damages make me feel better? No.

Years later, people continued to ask me why I hadn't sued the surgeon, so I decided to find out if I would have had a case. I spoke with a medical malpractice attorney. "No" was her immediate response. No, because negligence was difficult to prove. No, because we couldn't prove he'd caused irrevocable harm. Meaning, no, because I hadn't been dismembered or killed.

I didn't die on the operating room table. But Dr. B's mistake—or the mistake that was yet to come—may in fact increase my risk of metastasis and lead to my early demise.

Here's why: most cancers are insidious, sneaky, and not forgiving of physician error. Therefore, mistakes in cancer care can shorten patients' lives. In my case, there are a few possibilities. One is that Dr. B disturbed the tumor, that the "minuscule" amounts of cancer reported by the pathologist were shards of the original tumor dislodged by Dr. B's knife. Cutting the tumor could have released millions of cancer cells into my body. My cancer had tested positive for the hormone estrogen. Estrogen-positive breast cancer is notorious for silently re-seeding in distant tissue and lying dormant for ten, fifteen, or twenty years before it returns as stage 4 metastatic disease, which would kill me. But it is a moot point because no one will be able to connect the dots between my botched surgery and a future metastasis. Even when caught early and even when there is no family history, breast cancer spreads nearly 30 percent of the time. If mine were to spread, there is no way to know if the mistake played a role or not. Cancer is wily that way.

Later, when pressed, Dr. B did apologize again, but he never used the word *mistake*. Weeks later Mary and I found out my case was presented at the hospital's weekly morbidity and mortality meeting where physicians reviewed and discussed the week's mistakes and identified changes in policy or protocol that might prevent repetition of the error. But Mary and I were not privy to the conversation. We contacted the hospital's ombudsman, but he said there was nothing he could do for us.

From our perspective, the hospital made the mistake disappear. In my medical record, the do-over surgery was labeled a re-excision, a reopening of the surgical site to remove a wider margin of tissue. Up to 30 percent of all breast cancer surgeries necessitate a re-excision. So, on paper, my case does not look out of the ordinary.

The following month, in our mailbox, paperwork arrived showing that my health insurance company had paid to correct Dr. B's mistake. He had claimed his full surgical fee, twice. Spitting mad, I phoned my insurance company to explain that it was Dr. B's error and that he should have to pay for it. But the beleaguered-sounding customer service rep told me it wasn't the company's job to parse what was or wasn't a mistake. If the billing made sense, they paid it. And that's how the mistake was recast as "going back for more tissue." As if the mistake never happened. Erased.

CHAPTER 14

Winter turned to spring. Temperatures rose and layers of clothing were shed. Since the surgeries, I'd hidden my flat chest behind bulky sweaters, sweatshirts, and coats. Before the surgery, I'd worn light, neutral colors. Shades of white, beige, and brown that complemented my light brown hair and my skin's yellow undertones. But my post-surgery wardrobe was dominated by black and charcoal, colors matching my bereft mood.

Years later, I would find online groups filled with women who'd chosen to go flat. Groups where women traded fashion tips and posted pictures of themselves in their favorite outfits. But, in 2009, the only tips I found were for women who'd had a single mastectomy and were dressing in hopes of blurring the fact they had only one breast. The advice was to wear small, busy patterns, such as zigzags, houndstooth, even tie-dye. I'd never been one for prints, but I began to buy shirts with polka dots, stripes, and animal prints. The more I tried to hide my chest, the more I lost sight of myself.

On a warm Saturday, a day when the windows were open to spring breezes tinged with lilac, I grabbed paper grocery bags from the kitchen and headed upstairs to purge my closet of clothes built for bodies with breasts. Material meant to cover breasts gathered and bunched on my flat chest like a pair of wilted corsages. Into the bags went dresses and blouses with darts. A stack of white T-shirts, lest my scars be seen. And any shirt or sweater with a V-neck.

Mary popped her head in the bedroom and looked at a plum-colored dress crumpled in one of the paper bags. "But sweetie, you love that dress," she said. "Why are you getting rid of it?"

"It doesn't fit the situation." I pointed to my chest and made a sweeping circle. The muscled young star from the reality show Jersey Shore referred to his six-pack abs as "the situation," and I'd adopted the phrase.

She paused. I braced myself for what was going to be her fix-it strategy. But instead, she bobbed her head, said "gotcha," and ducked into her office.

An hour later, three bulging grocery bags sat next to the bedroom door. It was time to tackle the hardest part. Inside the bottom drawer of a walnut dresser with water-stained legs, a cast-off from the Peterson Palace, were my bras. The cotton everyday white, the black lace for special occasions, the strapless. Folding each one with care, I nested one cup behind the other, tucking in the straps.

Bras and I had a complicated history. Like many women, I sometimes resented the constriction, especially in the summer when the extra material and elastic collected sweat and smells. After college I went through a bra-free stage, refusing to don one even during a hot and dusty week I spent hiking in New Mexico with my mother. A fact she surely noticed as twenty-something me bounced along the trails in my thin cotton T-shirt but she thankfully didn't comment on.

Only in my late twenties and early thirties, while living in San Francisco, did I start to see the trappings of normative femininity as optional adornments to pick and choose. Seeing bras as optional, rather than required, allowed me space to experiment. I learned that bras can flatter as well as contain. Tease and tantalize. The mere sight of a bra strap was enough to get the imagination going. Sometimes, I would perform a strip tease for Mary until nothing was left but a black lace bra and skimpy underwear. The mood was playful and sexy. I loved feeling Mary's anticipation grow as I slid one bra strap off, and then another. Now, as the bras went into the bags destined for the Goodwill,

I couldn't help but wonder if Mary's eyes would ever roam hungrily over my body again.

The next doctor's appointment worth mentioning was the first with my big-shot oncologist, Dr. S. It was a month after my double mastectomy when Mary and I went back to the Simon Cancer Center to meet the oncologist whose advice would guide the next years of my life.

This was new territory. As a women's health journalist, my breast cancer assignments usually dealt with the pros and cons of various screening measures, like mammography and self-breast exam. When I was given assignments about the disease, the topic was often superficial and surgical, lumpectomy versus mastectomy. Few articles ever dealt with chemotherapy and even fewer mentioned hormone therapy, even though two out of three breast cancer patients cope with this life-changing treatment for five to ten years after surgery. That means millions of women are living post–breast cancer lives and enduring up to a decade of hormonal suppression, with the potential for considerable side effects, but no one—not even women's magazines—ever acknowledges or addresses it.

Dr. B had assured me I wouldn't need either chemo or radiation, but he wasn't an oncologist. Dr. S would have the final say. He would also have the results of my Oncotype test, a means of measuring the aggressiveness of my tumor. If the tumor looked to be particularly nasty, meaning more likely to spread, he'd recommend chemotherapy.

Chemotherapy sounded like a drastic measure. Chemo was for sick people. I'd heard it could do lasting and permanent damage to the body, causing nerve damage in the hands and feet, but my biggest fear by far was chemo-brain, the cognitive impairment so common among cancer survivors. I'd heard the symptoms—fuzziness, memory loss, and inability to concentrate—could linger for years. And, for some people, it could be permanent.

The thought of voluntarily signing on to a drug therapy that might permanently damage my brain made me sick with fear. What if I lost my ability to write? Writing was not just my career, it was how I processed information, how I made sense of the world. Even worse, what if I lost my ability to connect with Mary? Mary was a rigorous and out-loud thinker. I was a deeply curious listener and, thanks to my day job, an excellent asker of questions. But what if chemo left me unable to grasp the nuances of her intellectual work? Unable to follow the complexities of her mind and the academic world she occupied? Would she still love me if I couldn't think as clearly?

Finding myself back in this sewn-together building where the mistake had been made, where Mary and I had raced through the long, cold corridors to the mammography center, where we had confronted Dr. B about his mistake made my knees shake and my breath quicken. To pass the time, Mary had tucked a deck of playing cards into her backpack. We were in the midst of a rousing game of Egyptian Rat Screw, a card game I adored for its fast-moving pace and high-drama slapping of cards, when the knock came on the exam room door.

What I knew about Dr. S: he was president-elect of the American Society of Clinical Oncology and led the development of nationwide clinical trials in breast cancer. He was the most senior oncologist on staff and had come highly recommended by everyone we'd asked.

Things that surprised me about Dr. S: he had bushy eyebrows, a high forehead, tufted hair, and round glasses. He chuckled a lot, and when he did it was a subtle "heh . . . heh," his shoulders bouncing up and down in rhythm with his chortles. If Jim Henson had made an oncologist Muppet, it would have looked exactly like Dr. S.

Because my BRCA results were negative and my Oncotype score was middle-of-the-road, he said, "Chemotherapy would be overkill. I wouldn't recommend it." I could have kissed him.

Then he moved on to the estrogen problem. My tumor had tested 98 percent estrogen positive, meaning the sex hormone acted on my cancer like Miracle-Gro. He explained the standard of care for women in my shoes was five to seven years of Tamoxifen. The drug was the frontline treatment for early-stage, estrogen-positive breast cancer. Tamoxifen was supposed to block estrogen from reaching my breast tissue. I knew enough about Tamoxifen to know it was the safest and best-studied breast cancer preventative on the market. When he told me the drug would lower my odds of recurrence by fifty percent, I signed on with the optimism of the uninitiated.

Six weeks after my surgeries, I went back to teaching yoga. Since my cancer diagnosis in January, my life had been hijacked by tests, procedures, and surgeries. Fear and anxiety had distanced me from my body. Now that the worst was over, I needed to begin the process of easing back into myself.

The lobby of the yoga studio was hushed and cool. Dozens of wooden cubbies waited for the shoes, keys, and phones of students who would fill the space in the next few hours. I slipped my flip-flops off and padded across the faux-hardwood floor. The unmistakable scent of tea tree oil hung in the air. I strolled to the front of the room and unrolled the grassy green tongue of my mat against the honey-hued floor.

Kneeling on my yoga mat, my hips sinking back to my heels, my forehead resting on the floor. Child's Pose was a place to center my breath, to compose myself. But all I could feel was the empty space between my chest and thighs where my breasts had been. Swallowing hard, I willed myself not to cry.

Even nine years later, as I write this, the feeling of being breastless is hard to describe. The closest comparison I can draw is a Looney Tunes cartoon episode where Wile E. Coyote is shot through the chest with a canon—a perfect circle of emptiness—a violent window through which blue sky and billowy white clouds can be seen. A porthole of clarity and loss. Back in the darkened yoga studio, my forehead pressed to my mat with its faint scent of rubber and sweat, the studio door squeaked as the first student entered. It was time to teach.

For the next hour, I taught with my back to the wall of mirrors at the front of the room, determined to resist the pull of my reflection, fearing it would unravel my shaky confidence. Unable to wear any of my old yoga tops because the elastic put too much pressure on my still-healing surgical sites, I'd settled for a soft, stretchy black tank top. The thin material clung to my unevenly contoured chest like a second skin. A less stubborn person might have opted for prostheses. And, if I'd owned a pair, maybe I would have relented. But I didn't. It was breast-less or bust. And, wow, how much I missed my winter layers.

After class, two students pulled me aside. They had a friend who'd just been through breast cancer surgery. "Uh . . . we heard your class might be the best place to bring her." My stomach lurched. I wanted to blurt, "NO!" I barely had my own shit together. There was no way I could hold it together for someone else.

"Yes, yes of course," I said instead, pulling on my sweater and drawing it across my flat chest. "Tell her she's more than welcome."

The following Wednesday evening they were back with a tall, thin woman, her bald head wrapped in a red bandana. Georgia was a professor at the University. She'd been diagnosed with stage 2 breast cancer and was going through chemotherapy. Unlike me, she'd decided to reconstruct. In the coming year, we became fast friends and she would share with me how much she loved her new body. Our friend-ship helped me understand not only why women choose to reconstruct but also what an equally powerful expression of self-love and accep-tance it can be. But that night, she was asking me if she could do yoga with tissue expanders in her chest. I gave her modifications for poses that might be challenging and told her a little about my own situation. As we talked, Georgia deadpanned about her bald head and the tissue expanders. Her smile was kind and her sense of humor was wicked. Dark humor had saved me in the early days of my diagnosis, when

Mary brought home the wind-up boobs and friends gave my breasts a bon voyage with decorated boob cupcakes. But I'd struggled to find any humor these past few weeks. In that moment, as yoga class was about to start, it was all I could do not to wrap my arms around her. This new member of my tribe.

Later that month, Mary and I hired a pet sitter. We packed the car with beach towels, sunscreen, books, and snacks and drove north toward Lake Michigan. The sky was Crayola-blue and the dusty-green corn was high, its yellow silk draped like so many mortarboard tassels.

One of Mary's secret skills was making music mixes. In our ten years together, she'd made me more than a dozen mixed CDs that I listened to on endless loops in the car. Today she surprised me with a road-trip CD, and we giggled ourselves silly by singing everything from Beyonce's "Put a Ring on It" to "Boom Boom Pow" by the Black Eyed Peas, and the last song on the CD, Ingrid Michaelson's "Be OK ." Every time Ingrid sang the saccharine but irresistible refrain "I just want to feel today, feel today, feel today, feel something today," my eyes squeezed shut in hopes of willing it into reality. I so wanted to put cancer behind me, to move on. To be okay.

Mary's window was down, her hair was batting at her glasses. She was singing and drumming her fingers on the steering wheel. She caught me looking at her, grinned, and squeezed my hand. I looked out the window, inhaled the sunshine, and belted out the refrain. As the afternoon wore on, rolling cornfields gave way to sand dunes and scraggly pines as northern Indiana gave way to southern Michigan.

The sun was still up when we pulled into the Lake Shore Resort in Saugatuck, Michigan, five hours from home. We registered and parked in front of the door to our room. The motel was a neat-as-a-pin operation. Colorful flower beds, neatly trimmed grass, freshly painted bungalow-style rooms. It was one of the few hotels or motels that faced the lake. Mary propped open the door to our room and unloaded the car. Then we made a quick plan to change and go across the street to the beach to catch the sunset. Within minutes Mary was in her two-piece and pacing the room. With or without breasts, I always took longer to get ready.

"You go. I'll catch up," I said.

"You sure?"

"Absolutely. Grab a beach chair for me."

With that she was gone. The room felt still. My shoulders dropped. My jaw loosened. I'd always had a deep need for quiet, alone time, but since the surgery, my desire for privacy, especially when changing clothes, was an unwelcome visitor. Whereas I'd never thought twice about being naked in front of Mary before, my new reflex was to turn my back to her whenever we changed clothes. Try as I might, I could not stand in front of her naked. The pothole of my chest. The round-ness of my belly. It was not okay. At least, not yet.

I pulled my bathing suit out of my overnight bag and closed myself in the bathroom. Last month, I'd bought a new bathing suit from Title 9, a women's sportswear company. The new suit was a tankini, meaning it had bikini-style bottoms and a top that resembled the tank tops I wore to yoga. The suit had a Hawaiian motif—white and green hibiscus flowers on a navy-blue background. My hope was that the pattern would distract people from seeing my flat chest. The old me had a closet full of solids. The new me wore groovy patterns with bold prints designed to inflict visual confusion.

Under the bluish light of the motel bathroom, off came the flip-flops and the travel clothes. A blast of refrigerated air from the room's noisy AC unit triggered goosebumps on my arms and legs, and I crossed my arm in front of my chest for warmth. That was the moment when I realized that my days of nipping were over. No breasts meant no nipples, meaning no embarrassing displays under thin summer shirts. There were so few perks to being breast-less, I chalked it up as a win.

I tugged the bikini bottom up and into place, cinched the white drawstring, and paused. The tank top would be more challenging. I gathered the slick material in my hands, ducked my head into the floral arrangement, and pulled the shelf bra's tight elastic band down across my ribs. Like most women's suits, the tankini has a built-in shelf bra to cover and support the wearer's breasts. But, on my chest, the lining bunched and gathered. I pulled the suit's fabric away from my body with one hand while reaching inside with the other, trying to smooth the extra material down. Then I adjusted both shoulder straps and tugged at the hem. The suit was on. I looked at my reflection in the mirror over the sink.

My body flinched.

My chest was flat.

Very flat.

Flatter than flat.

Concave.

I tugged and pulled at the tank top some more. The elastic was so tight I couldn't take a full breath. Or was it my nerves?

Well, Catherine, this is what you've got to work with. If you ever want to swim again, you've got to get over it.

I'd taken to giving myself pep talks.

I squared my shoulders to the mirror, lengthened my spine, and adjusted the straps. Maybe I would pass as a flat-chested woman.

Wrapping my terrycloth orange beach towel around my waist, I plopped a wide-brimmed hat on my head, shouldered my tote bag, and marched across the street to the beach.

"Cute suit!" said Mary.

On the beach that weekend, I snuck looks at people's faces to see if they were believing my ruse. But no one gave me or my flat chest a second look. And something else happened, too. For years, Mary and I had fallen asleep spooning, me on the outside, her on the inside. That weekend, for the first time since my surgery, I pressed my slate-clean chest against the warmth of her back, my arm draped around her body. As I drifted off, my hand grazed her breasts and, in the liminal space between wakefulness and sleep, the boundaries between our bodies blurred. Breasts became abundant once more, as did curves and flesh, melded together by the warmth of bodies, soft murmurings, and caresses.

CHAPTER 15

By late July, a curtain of humidity hung across central Indiana. On campus, as the mercury crept toward ninety, clothes came off and breasts came out. They bounced along in bikini tops. They held up tube tops. They peeked out from behind sundresses. How I hated living in a college town where ninety percent of the population was young and perky.

It was near dusk on the day when Lorraine saw me stooped over and pulling weeds in my front yard. She crossed the street and waved. Standing up, I arched my back hoping for a crack or two. My body ached from my single-minded focus of ridding my yard of crab grass, dandelions, and Virginia creeper.

An hour ago, eager to get outside before daylight faded, I'd pulled on a maroon T-shirt badly shrunken from too many dryer cycles. *No one will see me, it doesn't matter*, I'd thought. Now, not only was the T-shirt embarrassingly tight, but there was a v-shaped sweat stain on the front, like a giant arrow pointing to my flat chest. As Lorraine stepped into the yard, I tugged at the shirt, tenting it away from my body so the contours of my chest wouldn't show.

Ugh. Why was I self-conscious in front of Lorraine? The one person in my orbit who understood?

But Lorraine didn't seem to notice. She was buzzing with energy from her latest trip, a three-day breast cancer walk in San Francisco. She and her sisters were regulars at various breast cancer walks around the country. Sometimes Lorraine walked and sometimes she volunteered behind the scenes, helping event organizers to coordinate meals, water, and shelter. She always came home bursting with stories and even more energy than usual.

Since the ill-fated dog walk, my envy of Lorraine's rah-rah attitude had morphed into appreciation. She told me stories about the breast cancer fund-raiser—the blisters, the tent-camping, and the speeches. In her tone, I heard how comforting it was for her to share a cause both personal and galvanizing with her sisters. Even though old me had been critical of such events, new me could imagine the intoxication of spending three days walking sixty miles with thousands of other women. A shared history and a shared purpose. I wondered if it was similar to the sense of connection and belonging I'd experienced in queer spaces.

But then her tone shifted to a lower register as she leaned toward me. For the first time, I noticed the gray streaks in her auburn hair and her deepening laugh lines.

"I think I finally understand how they feel," she said.

"Who?" I asked, flapping my shirt with one hand and slapping at a mosquito with the other. It was dusk. We'd need to go inside soon or risk bloodletting.

"Young women who look in the mirror and only see what's wrong."

My hands stopped fidgeting.

Had Lorraine sensed my self-consciousness about my shirt?

"You know," she said, "Like teenage girls who are really thin but they look in the mirror and see themselves as fat."

Whoa, this was not about me.

"Anorexia?" I asked.

"No, body dysmorphic disorder," she said.

"Oh."

Beads of sweat slid from my forehead into my eyebrows. I mopped my face with the back cuff of my garden glove. A mosquito whined in my ear.

"I don't know about you," she said, "but sometimes it's hard to look in the mirror. I never understood before, you know, how someone could hate the way her body looked but, well, I think I get it. I have a lot more compassion for those girls."

Inside the house, Emma was barking. She'd heard me talking to someone and couldn't tell if it was a neighbor or one of the guys who ambled past our house at dinnertime on their way to the nearby Community Kitchen, Bloomington's popular soup kitchen. If I was weeding near the sidewalk, the men would sometimes jeer at me or ask for money. If Emma was in the yard, the men never bothered me.

"I know what you mean. It sucks," I said.

I didn't know what else to say. I was no stranger to those feelings, but I never guessed Lorraine with her unbridled laugh and "boobs in a drawer" boasts ever felt that way.

And then her eyes snapped back to mine and she smiled. "Well, you better get inside and tell that dog of yours to settle down. Give her a pat for me, okay?"

"Yeah, will do."

The next time I saw Lorraine, she was laughing and race-walking behind her rambunctious dogs. We never mentioned the conversation again.

A week later, Dr. B glided into the exam room and offered us handshakes, smiles, and generic pleasantries. The man who'd dropped his surgeon's bravado three months ago to apologize and ask for our understanding was nowhere to be seen. Mary and I exchanged glances as if thinking the same thing.

Did he even remember?

How could he forget?

It was six weeks after the fuck-up, and Mary and I were back in Indianapolis for my three-month follow-up. Knowing the stakes were low—a simple follow-up or two and then I'd be released from his care—I'd decided not to go to the trouble of finding a new surgeon. And, besides, Dr. B had clearly been shaken by the mistake. Surely his ego had been checked.

He opened the front of my light-blue hospital gown to examine the newly healed scars. He leaned his anvil head closer, the smell of turkey sandwich rising from his breath. The roll of his jowls poured over the crisp collar of his button-down shirt. His tongue clicked behind his teeth, a sound I took to mean that he was pleased with the healing process.

My body tensed, expecting him to bring up the mistake, but he stuck to topics like the new book he was reading and "any plans for this weekend?"

Before stepping out the door, he dipped his chin, looked me in the eye, and said, "I thought you'd want to know I made a significant contribution in your name to the Young Survival Coalition." His hands were clasped, resting on his stomach. "It's a great organization. You should get to know it."

WTF?

So was that his definition of closure?

Cathy came in to schedule a follow-up appointment.

"Is there another surgeon in this practice who can pick up from here?" I asked.

"Of course," she said. "I totally understand."

Soon, Tamoxifen's side effects bubbled to the surface. First came fatigue and fuzzy thinking. Sitting at my desk, with a view of the garden—bees buzzing, flowers waving, words in my head flighty, like butterflies. Me chasing them. Pinning one, then two, to the page. Then came the hot flashes. The fiery furnace of my body belching hot air up through the collar of my shirt, making sweat bead on my forehead.

What took longer to surface was the slow drying up of tissues that needed estrogen to stay lubricated. One afternoon, Emma and I were walking home from the park. The sun baked the pavement. We began to climb the final hill leading up to the house, both of us panting. And that's when I felt it—a deep, painful twinge at the center of my being. My pace slowed. The pain continued. I stopped. The pain stopped. I started. The pain started.

Moving in slow motion, I lifted one knee, stuck out my leg, put my heel down, and rolled through the toe. Ouch. Emma lay down in a nearby patch of grass to observe my odd behavior. With each step, I zeroed in closer to the source of the pain, like searchers tracking the ping of a black box after a crash. I stopped when I realized where it was coming from. From a place I'd never felt this kind of pain before. It was as if the insides of my vagina had been replaced with sandpaper. The rough walls rubbed together as I walked. This was new. This was not okay. I tugged at the dog's leash. She lumbered to her feet and we tiptoed home.

Between the Tamoxifen and the double mastectomy, I wasn't feeling particularly sexy that summer. And the fact that I was married to a woman made the loss of my breasts both easier and harder to accept.

I'm embarrassed to admit that breasts are my favorite body part. An abundance of breasts is one of the best things about sleeping with women. When two women are naked in bed, breasts are everywhere. Billowy and soft. Sensual and round. Nipples erect at the slightest brush of lips or fingertips. An attraction to breasts may be the only thing I understand about straight men.

If I were married to a man, women's breasts would no longer have been a part of my daily landscape. Maybe I would have brushed my palms together, tsk-tsk, and said, "I'm done with those now." I might still see bare breasts in the changing room at the gym or swimming pool, but it wouldn't be every day, and it wouldn't be in the place where I was the most vulnerable, the place where I was struggling to come to terms with my new shape—the bedroom.

But that is so not my story.

I am married to a woman.

The fact that she has beautiful breasts fills me with pleasure and, when I'm least expecting, socks me in the gut.

The first time I saw Mary's breasts, we were in our late-twenties and making out on the futon in my studio apartment in San Francisco's Mission District. Her blue and red plaid short-sleeved shirt had snaps. The shirt was easy to remove, but the sports bra was more formidable. She sat upright, crossed her arms in front of her chest, and, in one graceful move, bowed her head, arched her back like a cat, and slithered out of the tight elastic. When I saw them tumble free of the sports bra, I'm pretty sure I let out a small gasp. They were beautiful. Teardropped shaped, sized in perfect proportion to her frame. They were plentiful and perky. They were everything my breasts were not. I liked my breasts, but they were the training-wheel versions of Mary's.

Before cancer, we'd always slept naked, steal appreciative glances at each other's bodies as we undressed. A sweet moment of vulnerability that often led to sex. Now I found myself turning my back to Mary as I changed for bed. I told myself that it was silly to feel self-conscious. She'd seen my chest at its worst—raw incisions, tubes sprouting from both sides.

What was my problem?

She assured me again and again that when she looked at my body she saw the shapeliness and strength of my legs, the rippling of lean muscle across my back, the graceful curve of my biceps. I didn't believe her. My eyes could only see what was missing.

One night, Mary was in bed reading and I was undressing with my back to her, as was my new habit. I stepped out of my jeans, lifted my shirt up and over my head, then reached for a simple black tank and slipped it on, pulling the bottom hem down over my scars. I closed the dresser drawer and turned around. Mary had lowered her book, her eyes on me.

"What?" I asked, a tightness constricting the back of my throat.

"Nothing," she said, starting to lift the book back up.

"What?" Even as I pressed her for an answer, I knew I didn't want to hear it. As long as we didn't talk about my body, the camisoles, and the scars, I could pretend my self-consciousness didn't affect her. We could pretend things were fine. But that wasn't Mary's way. Mary named things.

"I'm not bothered by the scars or the fact that you don't have breasts." Her words came slowly.

I braced myself for what was coming next.

A siren wailed as an ambulance sped past the house.

"It's just," she stalled. Her fingertips drummed softly on the paper cover of her book. "It's just . . . I loved how at home you were in your skin," she said. "That confidence you had in your body, the ease you felt . . . that's what I fell in love with. I never thought . . . well, I never thought you'd lose that."

My body hardened. I stalked to my side of the bed and yanked the covers back. I heard judgment in her voice. As if she was saying that if only I'd been a stronger, more confident person, I wouldn't have let the loss of my breasts devastate me. As if I'd let her down. I climbed into our bed, hugging my side of the mattress and facing the wall. "Easy for you to say," I seethed. "I never thought I'd lose that, either."

What I didn't say was that she was right. I'd lost something I didn't know I could lose—a comfort in my own skin.

Meanwhile, word of my diagnosis spread through my small network of editors in New York, and I was juggling several offers to write about breast cancer. I could hear the excitement in my editors' voices—who better to write about breast cancer than a women's health journalist who'd been through it! Many of the magazines had non-compete clauses in their contracts, meaning I couldn't write about breast cancer for more than one in any six-month period. I needed to choose wisely.

The problem was they wanted breezy articles about new medical discoveries in the fight against breast cancer, about mammograms saving women's lives, about foods that could prevent cancer. Before cancer, I would have easily taken any one of those assignments. But now everything looked different. Breast cancer was complicated. New discoveries for treating breast cancer were rare. Mammograms were attracting criticism for the number of false-positives they sparked and indolent cancers they found. And new double-blind studies were dispelling the notion that women could do much to prevent the disease. While weight gain and alcohol consumption caused upticks in risk, diet and exercise studies were disappointing failures.

Still, my editors weren't interested in my pitches about the disease's complexities and controversies. "Women want to feel good about their ability to outsmart breast cancer," more than one editor told me. And I knew the attention editors paid me would be fleeting. I was tempted to take the highest-paying assignment because my income had tanked in the months since my diagnosis.

But I couldn't do it. I couldn't go back to writing stories about the top ten cancer-preventing foods and the importance of yearly mammograms. So I took an assignment I knew I could write without compromise: a story for *Natural Health* about what to do when a friend is diagnosed with breast cancer. I interviewed a psychiatrist and a social worker, both of whom specialized in treating breast cancer patients, as well as a couple of survivors. My sources talked about the importance of providing a listening ear, not second-guessing your friend's treatment decisions, and not wondering aloud how your friend got breast cancer in the first place. It felt good to write a story that helped women support their friends who were going through treatment.

As much as I struggled to find my footing at work, Mary seemed to pick up right where she'd left off. Every day she'd jump out of bed, buzz out of the house, and boomerang back twelve hours later brimming with stories of students and colleagues, classes and meetings, office politics and academic minutia. Unfamiliar feelings of jealousy tugged at me whenever she left the house. I was envious of her clean break. That she had a part of her life uncontaminated by cancer. Once she stepped on campus, everything was right in her world. Friends, colleagues, students, even the physical space of her office . . . it all looked the same post-cancer as it had pre-cancer.

One night, as we sat at the yellow table eating the dinner I'd cooked while procrastinating finding new work, she told me about her day, about her students, and about a colleague whose husband had just been diagnosed with lung cancer.

I nodded, my spoon half-raised.

Her eyes met mine, the tone in her voice downshifted, "Wait. Are you crying?"

I sniffled and wiped the corner of my eye with my sleeve.

"No."

For the first time I had noticed how healthy she was, how full of life, full of promise, full of optimism about the future. The way her chestnut-brown hair didn't have a single strand of gray, the way her eyes danced when she was feeling good about her day at work, the way she seemed to have endless energy for life.

"You're not still thinking about your cancer, are you?"

A spark of anger flashed behind my eyes. "Are you serious?"

How could I not still be thinking about my fucking cancer?

Her look was equal parts disbelief and pity. For Mary, cancer was in her rearview mirror and she was pressing on the gas. But my engine had stalled. What's worse is that she hadn't noticed. I wanted to tell her that I was stuck in a bog of fear and anxiety, that I was terrified I didn't know if I could do my job anymore. Cancer had changed me in ways neither one of us understood.

CHAPTER 16

In the months since my surgery, I'd been content to pass as a small-busted woman. Before cancer, my clothes were an expression of myself. Now, whatever I wore was chosen with a single-purpose: hide the situation! My go-to tops were a tie-dyed T-shirt plucked off the clearance rack at Target, a brown camisole covered in a small white diamond print, and a stretchy beige-and-white checked pullover. None of them felt like me. But my experience as a queer woman had taught me that being me wasn't always safe. Safety was about passing as straight. Post-surgery, a deep part of my subconscious dusted off that skill—subverting my true self in lieu of what felt safe—and applied it to passing as a woman with breasts.

Dark colors and prints helped hide the situation but even my best cover-up efforts didn't protect me from curious stares. On several occasions, Mary and I were standing in line for a movie, waiting for a table at a restaurant, or walking down the street when people (usually men) would see me and do a double take, as if they'd mistaken me for a young man until they noticed the smoothness of my skin or the curve of my hips. The gaze could be curious or questioning, but more often than not it was tinged with anger, especially if Mary and I were holding hands. My sense was that people were thrown off balance when they couldn't instantly label me a man or a woman.

And there was something else. Some of my straight friends assumed going flat was an easier choice for me because of my queerness. They knew that some butch-identifying lesbians bound their breasts to achieve flatness. But what they couldn't know was that my breasts were a part of my queer-femme identity. That there was nothing easy about it.

My stomach churned as questions tumbled through my head. Is this really what I wanted for myself? After working so hard to come out of the closet as queer in my twenties, was I really going to let breast cancer put me back in? Did I want to spend my life wearing clothes I didn't like in hopes that I might pass as a small-breasted woman instead of risking people seeing me for who I was . . . a woman with a body shaped by cancer?

At nineteen, I'd fallen in love with a woman. Things we had in common: we both had boyfriends. We were raised Catholic. We were book nerds. And we were clueless about love. So clueless that we didn't notice the signs of infatuation—a desire to tell each other everything, to sit together at every meal, to study together on Friday nights instead of joining our sorority sisters at that weekend's frat party. But you know who did notice? The women of Kappa Delta. By Thanksgiving break we were called before a disciplinary committee made up of the sorority leadership. My relationship with Anne was platonic, but our sorority sisters accused us of being lesbians because we were inseparable. We were told the girls were uncomfortable sharing living quarters with us. A rebellious, independent thinker, I was asked to leave. Anne—warm, hilarious, and brilliant—was asked to stay. We both quit and moved off campus together. Within a few weeks, we realized we were in love. But our upbringing in the Catholic church, with its sinful view of homosexuality, combined with the shame and humiliation of being cast out of our housing landed us both in the closet. Inside our apartment, we were two college students in love. Outside of the apartment, we were best friends who'd been wronged by the campus Greek system. When friends and family visited, we'd make it look as if we slept in separate beds. When friends came over, we'd hide anything that suggested gayness. (Goodbye, *The Norton Anthology of Literature by Women!*)

In 1992, the summer after my junior year, I applied for and won a coveted internship through the American Society of Magazine Editors. The prestigious program brought fifty young journalism students to New York and sprinkled them in the offices of the most glamorous glossies in the City. Most of us spent the summer fact-checking, researching, and entry-level reporting. We lived together in a dorm at New York University. There were five other interns in my three-bedroom suite at NYU, and none of them knew I was queer. My experience of being kicked out of the sorority left me feeling scared and vulnerable, especially when sharing close quarters with straight women. Afraid of being found out, I declined invitations to go to parties, bars, and clubs and quickly developed a reputation as a misanthrope. So I explored the city solo and tiptoed up to the edge of the gay community. My heart raced as I crossed the threshold of A Different Light bookstore in Chelsea for the first time and later when I got close enough to the Pride March to see the neon-pink feather boas and feel the vibrating thump-thump-thump of dance music blasting from the colorful floats.

I'd been placed at *Fortune* magazine. Needless to say, this was not a great fit for me. One afternoon, a top editor saw me in the hallway and asked if I'd do him a favor. He was writing an opinion piece about the homosexual agenda. He needed a copy of the new children's book *Heather has Two Mommies* to support his argument. Would I go to Barnes and Noble and buy him a copy? I dragged my heels all the way down Sixth Avenue. I purchased the book and trudged back to the Time-Life Building. My hands shook as I handed him the book with the cartoon of two happy lesbians on the cover.

I didn't make peace with my sexuality until I moved to San Francisco in 1995. Seeing people freely experiment with gender and sexual expression gave me the room to explore femininity on my terms. For the first time, I saw that being a queer woman didn't mean having to choose between being a lipstick lesbian or a flannel-wearing butch. I adored dancing alongside the glorious femmes and strong butches at pop-up clubs, like Club Q and the Litter Box, and at the Elbo Room where we'd all crowd in to see Sister Spit. Over time, I discovered my own queer style. I started painting my toenails and stopped shaving my legs. I wore short skirts with clunky Doc Martens. I kept my hair short but left it soft and wispy around the edges. Feminine, graceful, and slightly butch, all at the same time. My femininity was a part of my queerness. By the time I met Mary in my late twenties, I was at home with my body and my sexuality. I dubbed myself a "slacker femme." In the 1990s, the gay community was re-appropriating the word *queer* and lesbians were casting off traditional butch/femme labels in exchange for monikers with fuzzier edges, like boi, baby dyke, and grrl. I didn't know it at the time but I was witnessing the early steps of the movement toward questioning the binaries that locked sexuality and gender into two tidy boxes.

Now, at age thirty-eight, my sense of self was shaken. I needed to relearn how to carry myself in the world, a task made harder still by not seeing other women who'd gone flat.

More than 250,000 women are diagnosed with breast cancer every year, and women foregoing reconstruction is not a new phenomenon. Historically, 25 percent of women who have a double mastectomy choose not to reconstruct, and 50 percent of women who undergo a single mastectomy stay flat on one side. Considering there are 2.5 million women alive today who've had breast cancer, that's a lot of cancer-afflicted boobs. Yet, for the most part, flat women are invisible to one another. Audre Lorde's lament in *The Cancer Journals* was relevant for me decades later: "Surrounded by other women day by day, all of whom appear to have two breasts, it is very difficult sometimes to remember that I AM NOT ALONE."

That fall in Indiana, I did not know yet that, in four years, Mary and I would be living in Boston. That I'd be riding the subway downtown. That the air would be thick with sweat, urine, and motor oil, and that when we rumbled to a stop at MGH, a thin, middle-aged woman in a lightweight, short-sleeve shirt would board. There would be something about her that catches my eye, even though dozens of people are jammed into the car. She would be confident and graceful, not wilted or coming undone like the rest of us. Give her a minute. I'd try not to stare, but I would anyway, at least until I see it, that thing that is invisible yet recognizable only to me—a slight concaveness to her chest, a lumpiness to her upper ribs. I'd see how she held herself—steady but with care—and I'd know. I'd smile at her, but she wouldn't see me, and it wouldn't matter. There would be two of us here.

Fast-forward six months to the first time I revisited a handstand, the pose that inspired me to go flat. I was headed to Lucy's hot yoga class. Her teaching style was confident and warm, compassionate and heartfelt, without being annoyingly pseudo-spiritual. She taught physically demanding poses but never pushed students into unsafe territory. Hers was the class where I felt most safe to explore my post-surgery body. Driving to the studio, scents of spring and new beginnings in the air, my body felt stronger than it had in a long time.

My surgery had taken place one year ago. One year since the mistake. One year without breasts. One year of taking a daily pill to prevent recurrence and hoping the doctors were right when they told me, "You're on the other side of this disease now. You won't hear from breast cancer again."

My confidence wobbled as I walked into the studio and unrolled my mat alongside fifteen young women in tiny yoga tops. Their long hair was swept back in neat pony tails. Their limbs toned and coltish. In the mirror at the front of the room, I caught a glimpse of a short-haired woman with a T-shirt fluttering across her chest, like a windless sail. I used to see myself as a confident woman who didn't care what other people thought. But that woman was nowhere to be seen. In her place was a person still reconfiguring herself from the ground up, still shaky in her post-cancer body.

An hour later, the class was sweaty from a series of standing poses when Lucy told us to find a space at the wall to practice handstands. I hesitated. My eyes shifted toward the door and then the small clock at the front of the room. Class was almost over. Sneaking out early would be easy. The noise of two dozen yoga students bustling and sliding their mats, water bottles, and props to the wall offered plenty of cover. Had I been cleared for handstands months ago? Yes. Had I tried the pose? No.

My self-talk sounded something like this: *I'm waiting for my body to fully heal.* But the reality was I was afraid I couldn't do the pose any longer. What if my muscles felt different? What if I wasn't strong enough? What if I couldn't trust my body after all? What if my decision to sacrifice my breasts in order to keep my muscles intact, to maintain the integrity and power of my back muscle, had been for nothing? Before cancer, standing on my hands was the closest I'd come to feeling invincible. What if cancer had robbed me of that, too?

My nerves settled. Lucy had a watchful eye on her students. Everyone was trying the pose, even beginners who were clearly nervous. Some students were already upside down, their legs skyward, pony tails pooling on mats beneath their heads, faces bright pink from the effort. No one was competing. No one would judge me if I tried and failed. I grabbed the corners of my green mat and dragged it over to a nearby wall. Kneeling down, I spread my palms flat against the rubber and rolled my shoulder blades down and back to align my arms.

The trick to upside-down yoga poses, like handstands and headstands, was to tap into the body's natural alignment, bones lining up one on top of the other—muscles engaged but not overworking. My knees lifted up and away from the floor, my body an upside-down V. I fixed my gaze between my hands. My back lengthened. I took a deep breath. My palms were sweaty. Unless I went up in the next few seconds, they'd be too slippery to kick up into the pose. I took a half-step forward with my right leg and kicked my left leg up. Both heels tapped against the wall. My heart raced. My body made the adjustments it knew how to make—lower ribs drew in, tailbone lengthened toward my heels, arms and shoulders steady and strong.

As I held the handstand, my lattisimus dorsi stabilized my spine, ribs, and upper arms. The powerful back muscle worked in ways I imagined would have been impossible had it been severed. My muscles harmonized in familiar ways, engaging, supporting, and stabilizing my pose. I felt the familiar adrenaline rush of being upside down. My leg muscles hugged in and up, my feet stretched to the sky. My body was strong and whole.

When discussing reconstruction post–breast cancer, plastic surgeons often say, "Most women want to feel whole." And by "whole," they mean breasted. To me, "whole" means freedom to inhabit my body without pain or discomfort, to feel strong enough to support myself physically and mentally. But medicine is myopic in its desire to return a woman's body to the shape it was before cancer—just maybe with bigger breasts and a tummy tuck. Pretty quickly, the definition of "whole" starts to drift into "better than before" territory, but no one has stopped to recalibrate the language. Few women are told about the 30 percent risk of serious complication because cancer's false sense of urgency makes all of that feel insignificant. Plus, plastic surgeons tell me they like being the "silver lining" of breast cancer care. Worth noting, too, is that plastic surgeons are trained to look at women's bodies with a male gaze. Even female plastic surgeons will say that—because textbooks are written by men and most of their medical school teachers are men—they've lost the ability to see women's bodies with a woman's gaze.

Afterward, I rested in Child's Pose surrounded by the bubbling energy and laughter of other students. My forehead was pressed into the pliant surface of my mat, my pulse thrumming. My heart was full and light. Every doubt I'd had about my decision had been wiped away. Regardless of what I looked like on the outside, on the inside my body's strength, power, and integration was a thing of beauty.

I would like to say my happily-ever-after happens now but that's not my story.

CHAPTER 17

Since my double mastectomy, the lentil-shaped mole on my chest had adopted a menacing new personality. The border, once smooth and harmless, had grown angry and jagged. The surface, once smooth and chocolate-chip brown, had turned a brindled mix of black, brown, and beige.

After breast cancer, a weird mole did not feel dire. A fly-at-the-picnic level of concern. Still, a year after my diagnosis, the young surgeon who'd taken over my follow-up exams after I transferred out of Dr. B's care saw that the mole had changed its shape and texture. She asked me to get it checked out.

"Is it an emergency?" asked the scheduler at the dermatology office. "Nah."

Three months later, the dermatologist, a small-boned older woman with thinning blonde hair and smooth cheeks, peered at the mole with her magnifying mirror. This was my mother's dermatologist in Louisville. She was smart, confident, and decisive. She suffered no fools but hadn't lost her compassion. Her face hovered inches from my chest. The soft hoods of her eyes sagged at the corners like weathered awnings, the only clue as to her true age, which had to be near seventy although she didn't look a day over fifty-five.

"Well, I don't like the looks of that one bit," she said. "That's coming off right now."

Her high heels punished the floor as she marched to the phone on the wall. She grabbed the receiver, instructed her assistant. Seconds later, a scalpel and a needle with a numbing agent appeared. "This will only burn a little," she said, right before she sunk the needle into my skin, an inch above my mastectomy incision. Minutes later she sliced the mole off with the scalpel. Surely she'd told me she'd send the mole to her pathology lab, but I was too busy thinking *sayonara!* to yet another body part. This time, it was just a nibble—a thimbleful of flesh. Had I remembered my last encounter with a pathology lab, I might not have been so nonchalant.

Back in Bloomington, my hands wiggled into a pair of blue garden gloves with green polka dots. Standing on the porch with my supplies, I tipped my face up to the sun. The breeze smelled like rain.

Beneath my jacket and under my sweater, in the space where the lentil had been, three black sutures tied together an inch-long sliver of angry flesh. The three knots formed an ellipsis. A blank space. A pause. As if to say, "To be continued . . ." A familiar, slippery ooze filled my gut.

Picking up a digging fork, I shook the spiders out of my gardening shoes. In the yard, the wet grass squished under my feet. A fresh stack of yard-waste bags sat on the porch. The best way I'd found to open the tall bags was to shimmy one over my head like a sheath dress, reach my arms up and slap the folds out of the bag to flare it open, then bend at the waist and back out of it. I performed this bag ritual a few times and got to work cutting, trimming, and raking dead leaves, over-grown stalks, and old growth. Soggy, spent foliage from the previous fall littered the flowerbeds. Heaps of spent daylilies. Tall sedum stalks with rust-colored canopies, bow-legged hydrangea branches topped with papery blooms that Mary called "old lady swim caps." Bag after paper bag grew heavy, their corpulent bottoms threatening to burst.

Two hours later, I peeled off my garden gloves, stepped out of my clogs, and retreated into the warmth of the house. The nuzzles of the dog. The stillness of my office. But the feeling of unease trailed me.

Later that day, the dermatologist's office called. A voice with a Southern drawl asked me to hold for the doctor. News requiring a doctor's delivery was a bad sign. But I assumed the worst-case scenario would be that the mole was a slow-growing skin cancer. That, I could handle.

"Catherine? Are you sitting down?"

Wow, doctors really said that.

I was in the same chair I'd been when Jana from St. Vincent's had called to tell me my core needle biopsy was positive. During that call, wafer-sized snowflakes had twirled to the ground. Now, in the yard below my window, a row of velvet-green peonies waved their pink buds like clenched fists.

From the doctor's tone, things were not good. Maybe my teenage sunbathing had caught up with me. My mother had always warned me to wear more sunscreen, but as a vain teenager, I liked how the summer sun turned my skin the color of brown sugar, my hair the color of flax. My sins had caught up with me and the dermatologist was handing down my penance. Uncapping a fine-pointed Sharpie, I searched my desktop for a yellow legal pad. No doubt there would be instructions on when to return to her office for a series of follow-up appointments, maybe a small procedure or two.

"Your biopsy was positive for breast cancer," she said.

The black tip of the pen hovered over the paper.

"I . . . I don't understand. It's not skin cancer?"

Static crinkled on the line.

"No. I'm sorry. It's breast cancer."

My elbows rested on the desk. Fatigue swept over me. My hand pressed the phone to my ear as if her use of the word *breast* in lieu of *skin* was a result of static on the line. A mistake. A slip of the tongue. But then she said it again, "breast cancer."

There must be a mistake.

A year ago, those words had struck me dumb. This time, I resisted them.

"It can't be breast cancer."

"It is," she assured me.

"But that makes no sense. I've had that mole for as long as I can remember."

"Are you sure?" she asked gently.

"Yes!" My voice was getting loud. "Maybe the mole was invaded by breast cancer. Can that happen?"

"No," she said. Her voice clear and calm. "That was not a mole. It was breast cancer."

I rocked back in my desk chair.

"You need to call your breast surgeon and oncologist," she said.

"But . . . they'll throw the book at me. Chemo. Radiation. Everything."

"Yes."

Beyond the window, a city bus deposited a handful of men on the corner. It was dinnertime at the Community Kitchen. Emma began to bark from the next room.

"Call your surgical oncologist's office right away. Tell them what's happened. Have them call me. I'll send the slides."

Her voice was small and tinny. "I'm so sorry."

I dialed Mary's number and told her the news.

"I'll be right there," she said.

People respond to bad news in different ways. With the first diagnosis, I'd crawled into bed. With the second, I started a to-do list.

A Midwestern summer was around the corner. A hot, humid affair. Mary hated mowing the lawn, so finding a lawn service went at the top of the page. My eyes shifted to the empty vegetable bed. It would need to stay fallow another year. Tending a garden would be out of the question for me. Then there was the fence I'd planned on mending and the window sills I'd hoped to scrape and paint. The kind of odd jobs I loved because they anchored me to both my body and my house, giving me a sense of accomplishment and a reason to be outside. *Find handyman* went on the to-do list. These jobs would need to be done by someone else, someone who didn't have cancer. Fifteen minutes later, a key clicked in the lock, and Emma barreled downstairs at full speed.

A breast cancer tumor can grow anywhere there is breast tissue. Breast tissue can be found as far north as the clavicle, as far south as the bottom ribs, and as far east and west as the longitudinal lines of the armpits. It can also be found at the surface of the skin in and around the chest. I would later find out that skin recurrence in breast cancer patients is not uncommon. Most likely, that's why my new surgeon's suspicions had been aroused.

What confounded me most was not that a lentil-sized dollop of breast cancer had been growing unnoticed on the surface of my skin for so long but that an internist, a general surgeon, three breast cancer surgeons, and, most recently, a dermatologist had seen the lesion and not recognized it for what it was—a second tumor.

CHAPTER 18

And now we've arrived here: the second diagnosis.

In hindsight, maybe seeing a general dermatologist hadn't been the best idea. My mother's dermatologist was excellent, but a doctor who treats dozens of skin complaints and conditions, everything from poison ivy to psoriasis to crow's feet, sees patients differently than a dermatologist who sees cancer patients all day, every day. Given the mole's location—one inch above where the cancerous lump had been growing—a dermatologist who specialized in cancer would have been a safer bet.

An oncological dermatologist might have recognized the mole as a potential outcropping of breast cancer and given it the respect it deserved. Physicians give breast cancer a wide berth. While there are many types of breast cancer, several are aggressive and many can be lethal. In general, great care is taken not to disturb the tumor. To inflict damage is to potentially unleash millions of cancer cells into the patient's body and heighten the risk of future metastasis.

Metastatic breast cancer is incurable. Once diagnosed, the average patient lives three years. Upward of forty thousand women die of metastatic breast cancer every year. Why one person's cancer spreads and another's does not is largely unknown, but one way to lower the odds is to remove a buffer of healthy tissue (margins) with the tumor. The problem was that two weeks ago, my dermatologist had sliced a breast cancer tumor off the surface of my skin as calmly as a home cook might carve a sprout off an Idaho russet. In essence, she'd given me a lumpectomy.

"Have you been taking the Tamoxifen?" asked Dr. B.

"Yes."

"Every day?"

"Yes."

"Are you sure?"

Hot bubbles of anger rose in my chest. I'd swallowed the damn Tamoxifen daily for a year. For months I'd been dealing with the side effects of low estrogen, fatigue, the fuzzy thinking, and the sandpaper. If anyone should have been asking questions, it was me.

"Yes, I'm sure." The air inside the familiar room at the Simon Cancer Center sizzled. The movement of doctors and nurses in and out of my room, usually efficient but plodding, was jazzed as if free shots of espresso were being handed out in the hallway.

Gone was everyone's breezy optimism, the intonations of "I've seen this before" and "don't worry, we've got you covered." Now the doctors' tones were lower, measured, curious. As in, "Well, isn't this interesting?" The nurses' voices were soft and pitiful, as in, "Oh dear."

Dr. B scanned the latest pathology report.

Yes, I'd gone back to him.

Let me explain. My new surgeon, Dr. B's replacement, was a young assistant professor in the medical school. In the year since the mistake, we'd seen each other twice. Attentive and astute, she was the one who had caught the changes in the mole, and for that I will always be grateful.

But compared to Dr. B's twenty-plus years of breast cancer surgery, the younger surgeon was a novice, less than ten years out of school. How would she perform? Had she seen a case like mine before? How was she in times of crisis?

If not her, then who? My mind had reeled at the memory of the time and energy it took to find referrals and interview surgeons, while worrying about whether or not a hospital and its staff would honor Mary's request to be with me in the recovery room. Whomever I chose would need access to my medical history, they would need to understand the scope of what I'd been through, and they needed to be able to coordinate care with my oncologist. But Dr. S worked solely with breast surgeons at IU Medical Center in Indianapolis. My options were narrowing.

Breast cancer specialists like to say that "diagnosis is not an emergency." That's because most breast cancers are slow-growing. By the time it's palpable, most lumps have been growing for up to a decade. Taking another few weeks to gather your wits, weigh your surgical options, and find a trustworthy doctor is the foundation upon which all future decisions will be built. This is not a time to rush.

With the first lump, I'd taken five weeks to make a series of careful decisions. During those weeks, I'd spent hours considering what kind of body I wanted to live in as I moved into my forties and (hopefully) beyond. Every woman values different things. I hesitate to even use the word *value* as it has been co-opted in a way that suggests morality. Some women value breasts. What I valued in my body was strength, ease, and symmetry. The slow-cooker of my brain offered this up only after I'd allowed the panic of the first two to three weeks to subside.

But now things were different. The mole had been cut off my body in a way that paid no heed to protocol. It felt important to have a breast cancer surgeon to finish the job. There was no time for deliberation.

I had picked up the phone and called Cathy, Dr. B's nurse.

The conversation went something like this:

Me: "It's back."

Cathy: "Can you come in on Friday?"

Me: "Yes."

Cathy: "See you at 9 a.m."

There is something else I am embarrassed to admit: I wanted all of my scars to match. For some bizarre reason, I still cared about the aesthetics of my chest. A surgeon's incision was his signature and Dr. B had a reputation for leaving clean lines. My incisions had healed well—two flat, pink lines. Nurses often told me they were the best mastectomy scars they'd ever seen. My chest may have looked like a hot mess to the casual observer, but it was my mess. I was protective of my body, my chest, my ordeal. As kooky as it sounds, I didn't want a new surgeon adding her signature to my page.

So Dr. B and I were together again. Nothing had changed, and everything had changed.

He washed his hands, stepped up to the table, and drew back my gown. A hospital gown never felt like much coverage until it was gone. Naked from the waist up, I sat on the padded table. My eyes drilled holes in the floor.

Dr. B was intimate with my body in ways I could not bear to dwell upon. His were the hands that cut off my breasts. His square hands, bulging jowl, shiny pate, and round, rimless glasses brought it all back. The fluorescent lights buzzed.

Mary sat on the visitor chair less than four feet away. I wanted her there, and I wanted her to leave. In the year since my mastectomies, I'd kept myself hidden. She'd seen glimpses of my chest, but she hadn't had a full-frontal view for a long time, not under the bright lights of an exam room. I wanted to crawl into a corner and hide.

To look at my chest is to see two three-inch-long mastectomy scars, plus a higher, shorter, newer scar on the left-hand side where the lentil had sat. (Funny that even now, as I write this, I feel an impulse to exaggerate the length of my scars to imply that my breasts were bigger than they were.) But to get a true sense of the distortion you have to feel my chest—flatten your palm against it, press your flesh into its contours. One of the first things you'll notice is that my skin feels stuck to my ribs in places, adhered like contact paper. Note how your fingers nestle between my ribs, as if sliding into the grooves between the black keys on a piano. The ribs on the left thrust forward slightly because of the mild curve of my spine.

Now the tips of Dr. B's fingers skimmed the edges of my newest scar, the place where the dermatologist had removed the mole.

My heart rattled against the bars of my ribs.

Everyone was quiet.

No one mentioned the obvious fuck-up.

Dr. B finished his physical exam but stayed in the room as Dr. S, my Muppet oncologist, squeezed through the door.

"Back so soon?" he quipped.

Not in the mood for pleasantries, I nodded.

Dr. S, Dr. B, and Mary discussed this new development. Soon, the three of them were volleying questions and speculations about the lentil.

Was it a recurrence?

Was it a second primary tumor?

Was it estrogen-positive?

If so, why did it become aggressive on Tamoxifen, a drug that should have defanged it?

The three of them noted how the new cancer appeared to be on the same vertical line as the original lump and, coincidentally, where my nipple had been. Could it have been on the mammary line? A third nipple?

Mary, a lover of primatology and logical explanations, sat up in her striped shirt and sweater vest, uncharacteristically engaged in the conversation. Her eyes were bright and focused.

"It's not a third nipple," I hissed. The words scattered to a far corner of the room. My vision tunneled. I peered out at Mary and the doctors from the back of my skull, watched as the three of them discussed the finer points of mammalian breast tissue. (For what it's worth: as fascinating as it was, the third-nipple theory was proven false.)

Everyone but me was distracted from the bigger questions at hand: Had my cancer spread? Did this mean it was metastatic? Or was it a recurrence? What did this mean for my odds of survival?

The short answer was that there were no answers.

First things first: a date was set for surgery. Dr. B would excise the site. Get clean margins. Dig down deep and take a small chunk of muscle from directly underneath where the lentil had been. Knowing my sensitivity to keeping my muscles intact, he assured me, "It won't impede the function of the muscle in any way."

"Fine," I said.

My tone was one of surrender. To care about my muscles now meant making another investment in a future that now seemed naively optimistic. A part of me was packing her bags for an early checkout from life.

As Dr. B opened the door to leave, he looked me in the eye and said, "Just one question, if I may—why me?"

He stood there with his saggy walrus mustache.

"Because I know you'll take care of it." I sounded like Tony Soprano ordering a hit. What I didn't say was that some part of me still trusted him. As messed up as it sounds, he still had a reputation as an excellent breast cancer surgeon, and the fact that he'd fucked up my surgery the first time felt like an insurance policy. Mine was not a case he'd forget. And, besides, he owed me one.

Cancer put our lives on hold. Again. Deadlines were extended. Classes were canceled, and days were lost to State Highway 37. A second breast cancer diagnosis in a woman under forty warranted more extensive and invasive tests than the first time around. A CT scan one day and a bone scan a week later would show if the cancer had spread beyond breast tissue. During my first bout with cancer, such tests were considered unnecessary. One test involved a potent amount of radiation and the other an injection of radioactive dye that precluded me from touching children for two days afterward. Before the second diagnosis, I would have balked at the risks, but we were past the luxury of hand-wringing about long-term side effects.

When we were home, Mary and I sat on the brown couch. The diagnosis sat between us like a stone. We didn't know how to alert our friends to the news that breast cancer had not been deterred by my lack of breasts.

What to do when the best-studied, most common, safest drug therapy for early-stage breast cancer fails? None of the doctors had mentioned that Tamoxifen could fail. But of course it could. Failure is always an option. Funny how that's so obvious in hindsight, but, at the time, I'd heard nothing but glowing reports about how Tamoxifen would cut my odds of a recurrence by half. To be fair, it does work for the majority of patients. In the world of medical statistics, you expect there to be outliers, you just never imagine you will be one of them.

Later, I asked my oncologist if he could have measured Tamoxifen's effectiveness in my body. A blood test to measure estrogen levels, per se, the way a cardiologist might track a patient's cholesterol to see if Crestor is working. He told me that measuring my blood hormone levels wouldn't work because Tamoxifen specifically targets estrogen receptors in breast tissue. Because I was premenopausal, a significant amount of estrogen was circling in my blood and latching onto receptors in other areas of my body. The only confirmation he had that estrogen was still reaching my breast tissue was if my cancer returned. He was as surprised as anyone by the lentil-shaped dab of breast cancer growing on my skin and the fact that it was estrogen-positive and had gotten bigger, as opposed to smaller, while I'd been on Tamoxifen. He'd tell me mine was the only such case he'd seen in thirty years of breast oncology.

Being an anomaly in the breast cancer world was not a good thing. With my first diagnosis, I'd taken comfort in the fact that millions of women had traveled down this road. For decades, scientists had collected and studied their data. Their legacy lit a path for me to follow. Illness had isolated me from the world of the healthy, but in the world of the sick, I was in good company. Now, thanks to the lentil, I'd gone off the grid. From here on out, every treatment decision would be guesswork.

The house descended into chaos. Emma wasn't walked. Dishes didn't get washed. Laundry piled up. Dust and pet hair covered every flat surface. My mother called and offered to pay for a cleaning service. "You know . . . until things get back to normal." In the past, we would have been too proud to accept help from my parents. Now we accepted the gift without hesitation.

So many gifts came our way in the following months that I lost track. The housecleaner Mary found for us insisted on discounting her fee. The young couple who owned the doggie daycare offered to keep Emma anytime, free of charge. Lucy offered to teach my yoga classes for as long as I needed. A staff member from Mary's department stopped by with a dozen Tupperware containers and briskly loaded two weeks' worth of dinners into our freezer. With my first diagnosis, I had struggled to accept help, confident that my role as a patient would be temporary. This time was different. The cancer was back and the future was hazy. I learned to accept what was given with gratitude and humility.

As we waited to find out if the cancer had spread, I holed up in my office with the dog for company. Late one afternoon, as the leaves of the giant maple rustled in the wind and the sky took on a green cast, my knees folded to the carpet and my fingers wrapped around the spine of a breast cancer reference book. Pulling it off the shelf and into my lap, I turned to the table of contents and ran my finger down the column until it landed on the word "metastatic." Kneeling on the scratchy carpet, the words that jumped out at me were that nearly 30 percent of women diagnosed with early stage breast cancer develop metastatic disease. Escaped breast cancer cells most often settle in the liver, lungs, brain, and bones. After diagnosis, the median survival of a person with metastatic breast cancer was three years.

The corners of the book dug into my thighs. I snapped the book shut and shoved it back on the shelf. Emma's soft snore drew me to the opposite corner of the room. Her plush bed, big enough for a toddler, took up most of the floor space. I rested my hand on her ribcage and slowed my breathing to match her relaxed rhythm. This is how we would get through the next days. Seeking comfort. Connecting in small ways. Finding calm and latching on.

The next week the doctor called. My CT and bone scans were clear. No signs of metastasis. The walls of the house exhaled. Mary, too, had been sucking in her breath, holding her body as if expecting blows to rain down from the sky. We didn't talk, shout, or whoop. We met at the brown couch. She wrapped her arms around me. My head rested on her shoulder. We stayed in that position as the sun set and the dog's muzzle nudged at our knees, her whines signaling that dinnertime had come and gone.

Clearing those two tests kept me on one side of the chasm that divides metastatic and non-metastatic breast cancer patients. *Metastasis* was not a word I'd have affixed to my medical record on that day, but nine years later, as I write this, it is never far from my thoughts. Breast cancer is a devilish disease. It can lie in wait for years. To say it bides its time may be to personify it beyond reason, but its ability to evade all radars unnerves me.

After the first diagnosis and treatment, I'd absorbed the forecast of full recovery given to me by all my doctors. But after the second diagnosis that kind of assurance was no longer possible, either for them to offer or for me to hear.

A few days later, Dr. B operated to remove a margin of tissue around and beneath where the lentil had sat. Beforehand, in the small pre-op room, he cleared his throat. "You'll be happy to know we instituted a new procedure."

In a haze of sedation, my eyes slid from his round glasses to the thick marker in his hand.

"Because of you," he continued, "I mean, because of your case, we started marking the area to be excised before the surgery. Your case will have a lasting legacy on the way medicine is practiced at this hospital."

He stepped toward me, pulled back the upper left corner of my hospital gown, and made a small "X" on the skin of my chest near the lentil's former resting spot. Maybe I should have been relieved that his mistake had prompted better hospital safety protocols or proud at having listened to my body's alarm and insisted on further testing after he'd declared the lump nothing but "fatty tissue"—but it was too little too late. Marking the tumor site was so simple, so basic. All I could think was, *Why weren't they doing that before?*

CHAPTER 19

After the outpatient surgery, Mary and I awaited the results of another Oncotype test. The genetic test later revealed that the second lump was a close sibling match, not an offshoot, of the first. To wit, they were fraternal twins. What importance to place on this information was difficult to discern. The test showed that the cancer, like the first, was middle-of-the-road aggressive. But chemotherapy was already on the menu, so the genetic results didn't offer much information. At my next appointment, Dr. S struggled to label my new lump. The word *recurrence* fell short as the lentil had sat on my chest all along. The phrases "local outcropping" and "second primary tumor" were also used.

Years later, when pressing one of my doctors on this question of whether or not the second lump was primary or secondary, he shook his head and said it didn't matter. His exact words escape me, but they were along the lines of cancer requiring an ecosystem to thrive, an ecosystem that was supported by breast tissue. The second tumor was simply another seed growing in the soil. The takeaway was I should worry less about the seeds and more about the soil.

On one point, my doctors agreed—whatever the second lump was, it was time for aggressive treatment. With my first bout of breast cancer, chemotherapy had sounded rash. Fearing it would dull my wit and rob me of my ability to write, I was happy when my doctor said it wasn't necessary. But, in the wake of a second diagnosis, medical consensus was in favor of chemotherapy. Now, my brain was the least of my worries. Dimwitted was better than dead.

We agreed to start chemotherapy as soon as possible and settled on a common therapy: four infusions of Cytoxan and Taxol three weeks apart. The next concern was my veins. The drugs were highly toxic and could do lasting damage to the veins of the arm. Dr. S recommended a medical device called a port. His nurse entered the room carrying a glossy, four-color package the size of a cereal box and lifted the lid, as if presenting me with a prize. Inside was a sample port. The device was the size of the plastic cap on a two-liter bottle of soda. Cancer was the ultimate disappearing act. Surgeons had chased cancer through my body with scalpels. Bits and pieces carved away—first my breasts, then the lump, and next went the lentil. The port was different. It would be the first addition in the face of so much subtraction. Agreeing to the port was an acquiescence to the disease, an uncomfortable reminder that my cancer had outmaneuvered my doctors. The time had come for stronger measures.

Port surgery took place the following week in Indianapolis. Once again, Dr. B did the surgery. The surgery was billed as "easy" and "routine," so Mary and I decided to go it alone. In the past, Mary had a friend or family member in the waiting room, someone to share the emotional weight. Today, after kissing me goodbye in the curtained-off pre-op area, she shouldered her backpack and headed back to the waiting room alone.

After the surgery, she maneuvered me through the hospital entrance. For a "routine surgery," it would be the first to leave me wobbly and unable to shake the clingy cobwebs of anesthesia. But I didn't know that yet. For now, we were flying down the highway toward home. On my lap was a sleek informational packet that came with the device, as if I'd just bought a new blender. The white, minimalist design was an obvious knock-off of an Apple product. Inside the box was a plastic key fob. On it, a bar code matched to the specific device inside me.

The flimsy, yellow-and-black tag slid onto my key ring next to the blue Kroger card, a pink CVS card, and a red YMCA membership fob. What would future archeologists make of these plastic tags we carried in the early twenty-first century, odd markers that tracked our movements, our consumption, and, now, my body's transmogrification?

Women going through breast cancer treatment posted their chemotherapy shopping lists online. The lists were specific and plentiful. Tips for everything from mouthwash to lozenges to wipes. (Thank you cancer ladies!) I collated, cross-matched, and highlighted. I pulled together the Mother of All lists, and Mary drove me to my happy place—Target.

Target's vast, white, aseptic sheen greeted me like an old friend. Mary steered the cart, a grown-up version of the red flyer wagon. Wandering among the aisles holding my list of chemo supplies was like back-to-school shopping. Except now, instead of my flustered mother foraging on the bottom shelf for the cheapest Mead notebooks and Trapper Keepers, Mary was chucking items into our basket with a spare-no-expense attitude. Ginger lozenges? Check. Purell? Check. Biotene mouthwash? Check. Into the cart went Kleenex, Tylenol, and Clorox wipes. In total, my chemo supplies added up to more than two hundred dollars.

It was spring 2010, but the economy was still reeling from the 2008 housing bust. University employees were in the midst of a salary freeze. Mary didn't say anything, but I knew she was worried about the bills headed our way. We were lucky to have health insurance, but we soon learned that each chemotherapy session cost six to seven thousand dollars for the infusion and an extra one thousand dollars for a drug to lower the odds of infection. Insurance covered 90 percent, but that still left us with seven hundred dollars out-of-pocket every three weeks. Our meager savings wouldn't last long.

Two weeks after my first round of chemo, I drove to the Indianapolis airport to pick up Beth. Back in January, before my second diagnosis, my two sisters and I had planned a "girls weekend" under the auspices of celebrating my mother's seventieth birthday. Her birthday wasn't until November, but we'd all wanted a warm-weather holiday and an excuse to get together without kids and partners.

My oncology nurses had taken great pains to schedule my chemotherapy around the trip. "It's important to have things to look forward to," they'd said.

Mary had chimed in, "It'll be great, it'll take your mind off things."

I suspected she secretly wanted me out of the house for a few days. God knows being around me was a downer. I would have jumped at the chance to take a vacation from myself. Mary was strapped in beside me on the cancer rollercoaster but without any of the support and attention that was lavished on me as the patient.

That afternoon, at the entrance to Terminal B, I stood on tiptoe to catch sight of my little sister. Throngs of summer travelers churned through the brand-new Indianapolis International Airport. Down the long corridor and through the crowd, a short, round woman waved at me. In my tiny fishbowl of suffering, I'd forgotten she was pregnant again. Of course, I'd known this. She'd called as soon as she'd gotten the news. But now she was in her second trimester and floating toward me in a bubble of radiance. Her eyes sparkling with glee, her curly hair bouncing, her belly round and ripe. All of my misgivings about the trip melted away.

Later that night, we convened at Lake Michigan with my mother and older sister who'd driven up separately from Louisville. Our plan for the next three days was to walk on the beach, swim in the motel pool, and read the stack of books we had each brought. The four of us were at our happiest when immersed in a good book with a refrigerator of snacks nearby.

On our first afternoon at the Lake, Beth and I straddled foam noodles in the hotel pool like giant toddlers. We made snarky jokes. Laughed. Rolled off our noodles and climbed back up for another ride.

As the sun melted into the horizon and the breeze cooled, I told her what it was like to lose my breasts, how scary it was to go through chemotherapy. How I feared Mary might have a nervous breakdown between caring for me and her high-pressure job.

Lamps in the motel rooms flickered on as Beth opened up about the miscarriages she'd had before my niece was born and how much she wanted this second baby. Each of us took the other's pain in stride. Not minimizing or comparing, but listening. Letting it wash over us as we bounced gently up and down in the heated water of the motel pool.

The next day, I got my period. Blood poured out of me for two days. My sisters emptied their luggage of pads and tampons, donating everything to my cause. Dr. S had warned me that chemotherapy might damage my ovaries and even send me into menopause, but no one mentioned that my ovaries might have a last hurrah.

I was ten years old when I got my first period. It was early December, a week before my eleventh birthday. I was in fourth grade. The first rays of winter sun were peeking into the window of the laundry room in the Peterson Palace. I stood before my mother, dressed in my Catholic school uniform—a white button-up shirt with the Peter Pan collar and a pleated green-and-navy plaid skirt with navy-blue knee socks. The toe of my sneaker sawed back and forth on the pea-green carpet. My cheeks were hot with embarrassment as I showed her my stained underwear.

"Looks like the curse," she said. "I'll show you what to do."

She led me into the powder room by the back door, opened the cabinet under the sink, and pulled out what appeared to be a foam hotdog bun. The Kotex was long and thin. One side had a white peel-off sticker. My mom pulled down my pink-flowered underwear and pressed the bun's sticky side to the inner lining. All morning at school, I sat frozen to my desk chair, terrified to stand up lest the boys notice the saddle under my skirt. When it was time to line up for lunch, I squeezed my legs together and pressed my back up against the cinder-block wall, praying I'd disappear.

For the next eighteen years, my period came every twenty-eight days and stayed for a full week. In fifth grade, I started babysitting and, for the first time, had real spending money. Soon after, I walked a mile to the SupeRx drugstore, bought a box of Playtex tampons, and taught myself how to use them. I also gave Beth the low-down before her period started so she wouldn't suffer the shame of the hotdog bun.

Before cancer, I appreciated estrogen. I could set my watch by my cycle, and I found the regularity comforting. After my first diagnosis, I was concerned about estrogen. My period came regularly on Tamoxifen, but I had to trust my oncologist when he said the drug was keeping the estrogen away from my remaining breast tissue.

Now I didn't know what to think about estrogen or about the ovaries that were responsible for making and releasing the hormone into my body. I'd deal with estrogen later. For now, the chemo drugs were damaging my ovaries, but they were not going down without a fight.

That weekend in Michigan, blood was everywhere. I once dated a performance artist who painted with her menstrual blood. (Remember, it was San Francisco in the mid-nineties.) I hadn't understood her choice of materials at the time, but if someone had handed me a canvas that weekend at Lake Michigan, I would have painted up a storm.

That same weekend, back in Bloomington, Mary was purchasing and setting up an elaborate new flat-screen TV in front of the brown couch. We'd dubbed the splurge chemo-vision, and whenever I broke away from my sisters and mom to call her, she was cursing and mumbling about pixels, wires, and high-def versus standard.

The television was Mary's freak-the-fuck-out moment, and she was letting herself go off the deep end. Some people shop for shoes, others obsess over handbags or power tools. Mary's weakness was electronics. The television was for her, but also for me—an olive branch maybe.

We'd had a fight after my last visit with Dr. S.

Two weeks earlier, at the end of a routine post-chemo check in, the oncologist had brought up the subject of an oophorectomy, the surgical removal of my ovaries. The room's overhead lights bounced off his glasses, so all I saw were his Muppet eyebrows wagging at me.

Surely I'd misheard him.

"Are you asking me if I want to have my ovaries removed?" I said.

"Yes, it's worth considering," he said.

"No way."

"But an oophorectomy would mean no more estrogen," said Mary.

Since the second diagnosis, she'd started asking more questions of my doctors. We'd spent hours talking in the car and at home, combing over my various options. But during doctor's visits, she let me take the lead, especially if surgery was up for discussion.

"Hell no," I said.

A look passed between Dr. S and Mary.

"But honey, it would make things so much easier," she said.

"Easier for who? No fucking way." My eyes welled with tears. "That shit is irreversible. Forget it."

The fight continued on the car ride home and bubbled up between us for several days afterward, but I refused to budge.

An oophorectomy would have thrust me headlong into menopause. Didn't she understand that surgical menopause would bring immediate hot flashes, night sweats, and brain fog? Didn't she get that there was no reversing an oophorectomy? That my body's chemistry, the delicate hormonal blend that influenced every cell in my body, would be irreversibly changed overnight?

I'd been willing to sacrifice my breasts in the name of lowering my odds of recurrence, but I wasn't willing to lose my ovaries, at least not until I'd exhausted every other option. It was bad enough not feeling like myself on the outside, I couldn't imagine not feeling like myself on the inside.

By the time I'd left for Michigan, Mary had backed down, but things between us were still tense. We didn't know this was the first of many times we'd have to weigh the potential but largely unknown benefit of more treatment against the preservation of my quality of life.

CHAPTER 20

When I got back home from Michigan, my hair was as lifeless as an old pelt. The month before, a hairstylist friend offered to shave it for me when I was ready. "I think it's time," said Mary. I agreed. Mary made a quick call and the friend drove straight over. I don't remember whose idea it was to take before and after photos.

In the before picture, Mary's arms are wrapped around my waist. Her head tilts to press our temples together. She smiles with her mouth closed, her face lit from within by a wellspring of optimism. Her eyes look into the lens without fear. She exudes strength and calm. In contrast, my body is stiff, my eyes distant. Look closely at my collarbone, and you'll see an unnatural rise, like a varicose vein but in a spot that makes no sense. That is the PIC line that connects my port and my artery. When I turn my head to the left, the tube tugs at me like an invisible rider.

In the after photo, Mary gives me a side-hug, her smile wider this time, her eyes radiating confidence. My head is shorn, more kiwi than Mr. Clean. My expression is flat, my eyes dull. A part of me was unhitching itself from my body's wagon.

The next afternoon, in the Kroger parking lot, I sat in the car waiting for Mary to do the grocery shopping. As chemo sapped more and more of my energy, she'd taken to goading me into the car just to get me out of the house. That's how I ended up sitting drowsily in the warm car. She'd left all the windows down but taken the keys.

Every minute or so, a puff of hot air brushed my cheek. My eyes closed against the sizzling glare of the sun reflecting off a sea of metal cars. My scalp felt prickly against the car's headrest. A lemon drop hockey-pucked around my mouth's metallic rink.

A car pulled into the adjacent parking space. My eyelid slid open. Dammit! It was our neighbor, a young guy who managed the local burrito shop, Laughing Planet. My butt slid toward the glove compartment as my hand fumbed for the side lever. FOMP! The seat went into a full recline. He was a sweet guy, but I wasn't ready to go public with my bald self.

Being sick in a small town gave people access to my underbelly, people I normally would not have invited to scratch it. Everyone we knew shopped at Bloomingfoods, ate at Michael's Uptown Cafe, and got caffeinated at Soma, a local coffee shop near campus outfitted with secondhand sofas, twinkle lights, and board games. With my first bout of breast cancer, my hair conferred privilege. I mixed and mingled amongst the healthy, and no one was the wiser. Back then I could choose who to tell and when to tell them. I was comfortable sharing my health status with friends, but less interested in telling the handyman who cleaned our gutters.

Soon enough, one day, the handyman spotted me resting on a bench on the outskirts of the farmers' market. His face turned ashen. *Please go away*, I telegraphed to him. He didn't get the message. Instead, he motored straight toward me. My panicked eyes searched the crowd for Mary who'd gone off in search of fresh corn. Seconds later, he materialized right in front of me.

"How are you?"

"Oh, well, not too bad." I wasn't going to just hand it to him.

I smiled and scanned the crowd of shoppers again, a universal sign of goodbye.

"So . . . are you feeling okay?" he persisted.

"Just a little cancer," I chirped.

Such awkward coming-out moments would punctuate my life for the next six months. The sad eyes, the pitying looks, the woman who followed me to my car in the Bloomingfoods parking lot to ask if I was in treatment and to tell me about her experience. The strangers who felt compelled to tell me about their mother/aunt/sister who had died of breast cancer.

Eventually, the cancer-killed-my-relative story happened so often I developed a shtick. As soon as someone launched into their sad story, I'd interrupt and say, "If this story doesn't have a happy ending, will you please stop telling it?" I felt like a bit of an asshole. I'd been raised to be polite, to listen and nod when someone else was talking. But two trips to Cancerland had left my emotions at flood stage. I'd lost my capacity for coddling. By stopping them early, I convinced myself I was doing a public service for cancer patients everywhere, but Mary suspected I was using my illness as an excuse to be rude. She was probably right.

The summer of 2010, each chemo session would lay me flat for five days. For the first five days after an infusion, I was unable to read, watch TV, or even think about moving. It was like being buried in sand. Five days of staring at the ceiling. Five days of rooting in the dark for words to string together to make a coherent thought. Five days of lying in bed listening to Mary in her office, as she attacked her keyboard and, every few minutes, forcefully cleared her throat. Whether the throat clearing was a tic or induced by gastric distress remains unclear, but it was an effective form of torture.

By day six, I was well enough to sit at my desk for an hour. With a smidge of concentration, my eyes focused on the screen and my brain formulated short sentences, mostly email replies. "Thank you for the card." "The flowers are beautiful." Anything beyond noun + verb + object was excruciating, deep-sea fishing without a net.

During this time, I found connection in online cancer forums, especially a group of a dozen or so breast cancer patients who'd all started chemo in June, same as me. As an introvert, I was born to lurk, but the people in this space eased me out of my shell. We shared tips on how to handle blocked ports, insensitive comments, weight-gain, and weight-loss; how to tie head scarves; and how to avoid the swine flu, which was raging that summer.

But the cancer groups were a breeding ground for anxiety. Barbara's breast cancer had metastasized to her lungs, Christy's surgical site was infected, Susan was hospitalized with pneumonia, Andrea's port was clogged, and Joy's husband had left her. My head spun with the pain and suffering my new friends endured, my sense of helplessness compounded by my growing awareness that an infection, a cold, or an accident could upend my own fragile health.

Mary would pop into my office with a question about dinner or the dog and catch me spinning about a woman's plight, projecting my own anxieties onto the screen. With a quivering voice, I'd tell her about Pat's rejected tissue transplant, Sue's repeated hospitalizations, and Kate's dying wish for her children.

"Honey, do you really think spending time in these groups is a good idea?" she'd ask.

"I'm not just walking away from these people when things get tough," I said, the rift between us widening. What did she know about this world? These people were my fellow inmates on Cancer Island. Mary was just my throat-clearing, keyboard-pounding warden.

"Please? At least for a while." Her voice was softer.

She just wanted me to stay calm and pliable because that would make her life easier. Fuck that. "I'll think about it," I said, turning back to the screen.

In July, Mary flew to Boston to secure a six-month rental for the following year. She'd been offered a fellowship at a research lab in Cambridge, Massachusetts. We'd be relocating from January to July 2011 and needed someplace to live, ideally an apartment close to her office with a landlord who wouldn't mind an eighty-pound dog.

When Mary had come to me with this idea six months prior, the old me would have ticked off a million reasons why we couldn't pack our bags and move to Massachusetts for six months. Who would take care of the house? What about my yoga classes? My family? My work? But new me didn't give a shit. Well, that's not giving new me much credit, is it? More likely she knew the details would work themselves out. Mary had proven herself more than capable of taking care of logistics. And whereas old me would have feared losing control, new me had awakened to the fact that control was an illusion.

While apartment hunting, Mary called me each afternoon with updates, her voice infused with the energy and enthusiasm of someone on the cusp of a fresh start. "Honey, you're going to love it here! The restaurants, the bookstores, the public transit. Hey, and I found the perfect apartment in Inman Square."

Slouching at my white desk, picking at a plate of scrambled eggs, seesaw-ing between hot flashes and chills, my fogged-in brain swept up all the positivity it could muster and blew it over the phone like pixie dust.

"A one-bedroom in Inman Square? That sounds great!"

Where the hell was that?

After we hung up, I sat hunched at the helm of my white ship-of-a-desk, zooming in and out on maps of Cambridge and Somerville, trying to find this elusive Inman Square. The closer I looked, the more confused I got. The dense city was a tangle of one-way streets, traffic circles, and six-way intersections.

Who'd ever heard of Somerville anyway?

Where was Inman Square in relation to Mary's office?

And what about Davis Square? Union Square? And Porter Square?

Somerville was only four square miles. How many Squares could there possibly be?

The phone rang. It was Georgia, the woman who'd come to my yoga class, the professor who'd been undergoing reconstruction after her own bout with breast cancer. She asked how I was feeling and if I wanted to go to a breast cancer support meeting with her that night.

"Sure." A spark of possibility flickered in my chest.

Mary would not approve, but she wasn't home, so who cared?

Mary knew that in-person breast cancer groups and I didn't get along. My outspoken introversion didn't win me any friends in these spaces. I found in-person breast cancer groups stilted, an unacknowledged hierarchy simmering beneath the pleasantries breast cancer patients exchanged with one another. My first encounter with the hierarchy wasn't in a group but in a chance meeting at the Bloomington Farmers' Market. A friend's sister was visiting from Canada and had been treated for breast cancer three years prior. As we'd stood among the stalls of tomatoes and rainbow chard, the woman peppered me with questions: At what stage was my disease diagnosed? How many lymph nodes were removed? Did I go through chemo? Radiation?

Her rapid-fire questions had caught me off guard. My answers were halting, hesitant. Her eyes sized me up, as if calculating the legitimacy of my case.

"So, you were just stage 1?"

"Um. Yes."

"You just had surgery? No chemo?"

"Right," I said, "I just had a double mastectomy."

As the word *just* left my mouth, I wanted to pull it back. I'd made it sound as if, by cutting off my breasts, I'd taken the easy way out.

What the hell was wrong with me?

I wanted to crawl under the nearest produce truck until the woman was back on Canadian soil. But it soon became clear to me that she wasn't an anomaly. Within the breast cancer community, people who'd gone through more treatment (rightly or wrongly) often felt more legitimate than those who'd gone through less treatment. On the spectrum of cancer patients, chemo was a dividing line between "fuck-you-up cancer" and "cancer-lite." Among those whose diseases progressed, more dividing lines, such as metastasis, seemed to appear. Initially, I didn't understand these divisions, but I learned to appreciate them as time went on.

The local breast cancer support group met at a failed-fast-food-outlet-turned-coffee-shop near the Target on the east side of town. Georgia met me in the parking lot at 7 p.m. that evening. In the time between my first and second diagnoses, she had finished treatment and completed her reconstruction. Her wavy reddish-brown hair was almost to her shoulders, and she wore her new curves with confidence and style. Still, nerves whisked my insides. She hadn't seen me bald and bicycle-rack thin. But her toothy grin put me at ease. We hugged, locked arms, and strode toward the door. Inside the cavernous stucco room, a woman waved at Georgia from across the room and motioned her over.

"You okay?" Georgia asked.

"Yeah, I'll be fine."

She squeezed my arm and walked away.

I pulled my shoulders back, held my bald head high, and smiled at the first person who made eye contact with me, a middle-aged woman with shaggy hair and thick glasses. I introduced myself, and soon we were sharing our stats.

Breast cancer survivors have a language for conveying the diagnostic details of their disease, a mixture of acronyms and shortcuts like ER-positive, HER2-negative, triple-negative, rads, mets, staging, nodes, and NED, which is short for *no evidence of disease*. In online breast cancer groups, many people listed these details in the signatures that automatically appeared at the end of every comment. Some signatures were fifteen lines deep and included details like surgery dates and drug therapy regimens. The whole thing was exhausting.

I told the shaggy-haired woman that I was in the middle of chemo and would undergo seven weeks of radiation in the fall. She nodded and told me she had DCIS, or ductal carcinoma in situ, also known as stage 0 breast cancer. Underneath my pasted-on smile, I thought:

Gimme a break. That's not cancer. I'll show you cancer.

Overnight, I'd been transformed into the breast cancer alpha dog I once loathed, growling with superiority and one-upmanship.

A white-haired woman in an aggressively purple tracksuit called the meeting to order. I want to say that I remember everything that came next, every name and face—Dottie's white coiffure, silver-rimmed glasses, skin weathered from seventy years of smiling and laughing, Beatrice's feathery laugh, gray perm, papery white skin—but I'd be lying.

All I remember was the well of loneliness that broke open inside of me as I looked around the restaurant and saw no one else in her thirties. Georgia, in her mid-forties, was the next-youngest person in the room. The majority of people present were in their sixties, seventies, and beyond. My biggest worries were how I was going to reclaim my sex life, my livelihood, and my ability to plan more than six months down the road.

Around the table, women discussed the crafting and marketing of pink-ribbon bracelets and sweatshirts. Even though it was only August, everyone was gearing up for Breast Cancer Awareness Month. Looking around the room, it was clear these women had fully embraced their identity as survivors. That wasn't something that interested me. Breast cancer had hijacked my life in my prime. I wanted to identify as a writer, a journalist, a yoga teacher, a queer woman, a feminist—anything but a pink-ribbon warrior. The future I wanted was one where my breast cancer history was the least interesting thing about me. If I got out of this alive, I swore I wouldn't give the disease anymore air time. As I stewed, a clipboard landed in front of me with a sign-up sheet for the pink-ribbon lanyards Sally's granddaughter was making.

I glanced across the long table at Georgia, wanting to catch her eye and give her a look that said, "Can you believe this lanyard bullshit?"

But she was laughing and smiling with a Betty-White-look-alike. Her acceptance of everyone here, regardless of age or pink-ribbon-politics, made me notice the stank of my bad attitude.

CHAPTER 21

A whoosh of heat and humidity greeted me in the lobby of the yoga studio. My stomach sickened at the smell of incense mixed with sweat. Thanks to chemo, my nose had become a sensitive tripwire for my gag reflex. Earlier that morning I'd snapped at Mary for wiping down the kitchen counter with a new cleaner. The label called the scent lemongrass and lavender, but to me it had reeked of rotting compost.

Students from the hot fusion class churned around the registration desk as I waited to sign in. The hot yoga studio was the biggest of the three studios and the most raucous—for a yoga studio that is. The hot room had walls the color of egg yolks, a thumping sound system, and a purring humidifier that created a monsoonlike climate minus the rain. In the winters, hot yoga offered me a reprieve from central Indiana's bone-chilling damp. My muscles would thaw from hard polymer to Silly Putty, and afterward my body would radiate heat like a wood stove. Before cancer, this was my second home. Now, the thought of a hot class made me queasy.

My new studio was the smaller studio next door, one with the soothing blue walls, dimmed lights, and a wall of shelves that held all matter of yoga props. Blankets, blocks, bolsters, and straps—everything necessary to support the body in relaxation or (as in my case) illness. After adding my name to the class roster, I ducked into the blue room and unrolled my mat near the wall. With each surgery, my body felt more feeble, more vulnerable. The wall offered protection and stability.

Lying on my mat with my eyes closed, a low-grade discomfort spanned from my heels, past my hips, and up to my shoulder blades. Since when was I uncomfortable lying flat on my back? Corpse pose was always the one pose I could do with ease. Nothing had changed. This was the same wood floor, the same yoga mat . . . then it hit me. What I was feeling was the weight of my bones against the floor. Each bony protrusion pressed into the wood laminate surface like brass knuckles. The contours of my body had been rubbed away by weight loss.

As the class started, the teacher encouraged us to be kind to our bodies, to shift our awareness inside. Under the dimmed lights, surrounded by women, I crept back into my body, ran my breath across its scars, examined its wounds. Toward the end of the class, in the twilight sleep of meditation, the teacher's voice instructed me to bring the flat of my hand to the center of my chest to feel the rise and fall of my breath. The movement was familiar. I'd done it thousands of times as a way to connect my breath to my body. But this time was different. When my palm landed on the bumpy landscape of my chest and felt the prominent outline of my ribs where my breasts used to be, it jolted back as if shocked by an electric fence.

In that moment, I wanted nothing more than to distance myself from what my body had become, to dive back into my underwater cave of denial. But I slid both hands onto my stomach instead, a safer and more neutral location from which to feel the undulation of the breath.

As my nerves settled, my hands registered an unexpected vibration. Pressing more firmly into the hollow of my belly, a drumbeat kicked back. It took me a few beats to recognize the forceful pulse of my aorta. The intensity of the blood pushing against the walls of my body's main artery shocked me. Everything about me looked fragile, malnourished, and sickly; so much so that I'd started to believe it. But under my hands was evidence of something else. An undeniable presence of life, strength, and persistence. The inner workings of my body were undeterred by four surgeries and multiple rounds of chemo. My aorta couldn't care less if I had breasts or hair. It didn't bright-side me or slap a pink ribbon on my forehead and label me a survivor. In my mind, its steady rhythm—*bum, ba-bum, ba-bum, ba-bum*—translated as "Don't worry, you've got this."

My body is sensitive to drugs, and chemo was no exception. Each infusion made me sicker as the toxins accumulated. *Infused* was a word I used to associate with teas and oils. But in Cancerland an infusion meant soaking the body in chemicals. Whenever I'd seek out my acupuncturist to help me manage the side effects, she'd make a voodoo doll of my body and, upon re-entering the room thirty minutes later, say, "Yep, smells like chemo." I smelled nothing, but the thought of my body emitting chemical-filled fumes was depressing as hell.

To measure the effects of chemo, I had to look no further than our walks with Emma. At the beginning of chemo, we stuck with our traditional two-mile, round-trip walk to Bryan Park, but at a slower pace. On especially sunny days, we'd add a mile or more by walking to the leafy Southdown neighborhood beyond the park boundary. There, we'd daydream about living in one of the adorable Arts and Crafts bungalows closer to campus, maybe one with a big backyard for a second dog.

After the second infusion, we put Emma in the car and Mary drove us to the edge of Bryan Park. There, we'd walk the paved sidewalk at the park's perimeter, which was just under a mile. A week after my third infusion, we drove to the park again. The sky was cornflower-blue, the trees lush as broccoli stalks, the dog eager to "run off her puppy ya yas," as we called them. We pulled into our usual spot and drank in the scene. Laughter rose from the playground. The smell of grilled hotdogs and hamburgers floated over from a party at one of the nearby picnic shelters. Students played frisbee on the grass. The dog hopped out of the car and shook so hard her lips flapped against her gums. Mary opened my car door and held out her hand, but when I took it and tried to follow her toward the walking path, my sludge-filled body refused to cooperate. My knees wilted, and I sank onto a bench. I was worn out. We'd gone thirty feet.

The cancer itself never caused me a single ache or pain; it was the treatment that was debilitating. Chemo's effects were often described as "accelerated aging." Before chemo, I'd been a vibrant, robust thirty-eight-year-old. Now, my muscles were atrophied, my skin was sallow, and my stamina was at rock bottom. Of course, my cancer would have pained me a great deal if it had been left untreated, but it was hard to remember that the chemo was helping, not harming, me. With every passing day, my previous identity as a healthy, independent person drifted further away.

All summer long, Mary and I argued about how many days I had to wait after chemo before I could drive. Sure, the drugs made my eyesight blurry and my judgment poor, but I considered myself safe to drive after four days, she said ten. We settled on seven. This meant that after every infusion, Mary schlepped me around Bloomington in her white 1997 Honda Accord.

Mary loved that car. She adored its faded blue interior, she fussed over the rust spot gnawing away at the tire well, and she didn't mind that the air-conditioning was broken. She didn't seem to notice that the car refused to accelerate past 30 MPH. And she was immune to the fact that it smelled like cat urine, an odor amplified by hot summer days. The cat piss was my fault. Years before, I'd let our cat roam free in the car on the way to the vet, and I was still paying for my mistake. Cat pee proved impossible to extract from upholstery. When the temperature climbed above eighty-five, the smell of ammonia from the backseat still made my eyes water.

That car encapsulated my summer of chemo. Mary patiently at the wheel, me clutching my stomach, head, or both as we puttered around to Bloomington's various healers. From the cranial sacral therapist, to the osteopath, to the acupuncturist. Mary dropping me off and picking me up as dutifully as any soccer mom. After each appointment, she'd look at me expectantly. "Did it help? Do you feel better?" I'd nod and report a lessening of a headache or an uptick in appetite, but in her daily repetition of hope-filled questions, I often heard an undercurrent of, "For god's sake, please tell me one of these yahoo therapies is working because your misery is driving me crazy!"

Something else gnawed at me, too. In our six years in Indiana, I'd never noticed the Advanced Pain Clinic near the mall where my acupuncturist worked or the Center for Wholism on the north side of town where a cranial sacral therapist restored my appetite, or the modest house near the highway where my cognitive behavioral therapist, Dr. Miracle (I am not even kidding), saw a steady stream of clients. Until then, I'd mostly moved through the world as a healthy person. Now I saw that if you flipped a town over, you'd see an alternate universe, a place dotted with unassuming office buildings where healers were easing the suffering of chronic illness. Breast cancer was my passport to this new place. Now that I had the documentation, I would always have a foot in both worlds. I want to say dual citizenship has made me a better person, but it's not that simple.

The experience of chemo could be distilled to the objects on my night-stand. The still life of an illness:

- A bottle of fancy sleep spritz Mary had brought me from a trip to Ann Arbor, Michigan. Such a sweet and unex-pected gift, I couldn't bring myself to use it.
- A homeopathic remedy my sister Ginny had sent. The label on the bottle of stale-tasting water suggested a few drops would diffuse feelings of panic and despair.
- A wooden cuticle stick.
- A paperback copy of Pema Chodron's *When Things Fall Apart*.

- A lipstick-sized blue plastic cylinder of Hyland's *Nux vomica*, a homeopathic remedy for nausea.
- A round tin of Badger Sleep Balm. Every night I took off the lid, circled the tip of my middle finger around the smooth, waxy surface, and swiped it across my lips. While pressing my lips together, I'd hear lip smacking from the other side of the bed, which was Mary's way of asking for some. I'd circle my finger again around the lavender-scented balm and stretch my arm out toward her face. She'd lift her mouth toward my outstretched finger and nuzzle her way to my fingertip, smearing the balm in the general vicinity of her lips, which made me giggle.

As my summer of chemo wore on, the drugs wooled my brain. If a task came to mind—call the doctor, refill a prescription, buy a birthday card—there was a fifteen-second window to write it down or else it would vaporize.

My freelancing career was now on life support, my capacity for work slipping more and more with each infusion. In the beginning, I'd block the first week following an infusion off my calendar, knowing my brain would be mush. The second week post-chemo was for interviews. At the end of the third week was my deadline. Then I'd begin the monthlong process all over again. That system worked in the beginning, but each chemo hangover hit me harder than the last, and my ability to write began to slip beyond reach. By the end, Mary was coaching me through my assignments one sentence at a time, fretting a path between her office and mine, setting a timer and checking on me every ten minutes to see if I'd managed to add a sentence to the Word document on my screen.

My final chemotherapy infusion was on Friday, August 27, 2010. I thought I'd feel jubilant afterward—or at least once the lethargy and wooziness passed. I expected to feel a sense of accomplishment. A sense that I'd endured the unendurable, that I'd earned a chemo badge to sew onto my survivor's sash. That I'd advanced to the next rank in the warped world of cancer promotion. But I didn't. I felt lost. A stranger in my body and unrecognizable in my relationship with Mary.

CHAPTER 22

Three weeks later, the morning of the Hoosiers Outrun Cancer 5K dawned crisp and bright. Hundreds of people packed into the parking lot of the Memorial Stadium just north of campus. I clung to Mary like a barnacle. My bald head quivered beneath its white bandana and my legs shivered in their baggy sweat pants. The previous day, we'd gone to Indianapolis for my port removal. The short surgery required general anesthesia. New me was cocky. She'd prepped for the trip to the operating room like old me would have prepared for a trip to the dentist, meaning not at all. Now my head was woozy and my right side, where the port had sat under my arm, was sore. I'd wanted to stay in bed that morning, but I didn't want to tell Mary and risk seeing a sanctimonious "I told you so" look.

Six weeks ago, when one of the yoga teachers at the studio had pulled me aside and asked if she could organize a team in my name, I'd panicked and said yes. Then I'd guilted Mary into doing it with me. "Can I sign you up, too?" I begged, the registration form up on my screen.

"Um. Yeah, no," she said.

"Puhleeease?" Groveling wasn't new to me. I didn't have the mental stamina to do the race alone. And cashing out some relationship currency felt better than reneging on a social obligation, even one to someone I barely knew. If the yoga studio was going to make me their cancer mascot, the least I could do was show up to play the part. Mary lifted her arms, palms face-up, in a WTF gesture. Her face screwed into a scowl. "Fine. Whatever," she said, dropping her arms and spinning on her heel.

That's how we ended up in a crowded parking lot at 9 a.m. on a Saturday morning in September. Me clinging like a parasite to Mary, neither of us happy about the situation. We were twenty-one months into the ordeal. Her foundation was solid, but her day-to-day patience was running thin. I didn't blame her. Cancer me was weepy, needy, and inarticulate. We could have both used a vacation from that sad sack and her everything-is-shit attitude. But that morning, there was no reprieve. Unable to pry ourselves from the misery of our dynamic, we stayed stuck. Mary was in silent-protest mode, a stance she reserved for special occasions. There would be no looking at me and no conversation. I was in needy-mode. My repeated entreaties to her elicited miserly one-word retorts. As we bobbed unhappily in the sea of cancer cheerleaders, I scanned the crowd for people from the yoga studio but, in my post-surgery haze, all the women swarming the staging area looked as ponytailed, lithe, and bedecked in athleisure-wear as the young person who'd recruited me.

Studying the crowd, I saw no other bald heads but I did see lots of families with matching T-shirts and handmade signs that said things like "We walk in memory of Nancy." My stomach sank to the pavement. How had I not known that people would be walking for those who'd died of the disease? If a crack had opened in the concrete, I would have crawled right in. We should leave. As I braced for the argument that would surely ensue once I asked Mary to reverse course and drive me home, the emcee took the stage. "WELL HELLLLL-LOOOOOOOOO, HOOOOOOOSIERS!!!!!!"

For the next ten minutes, his carnival barker's voice pummeled me with messages of hope and courage. Bodies pressed against me and strangers' shoes nudged the backs of my heels. The crowd was edging toward the rickety aluminum stage, toward the man with the microphone, toward the whoops and hollers about kicking cancer's ass and showing it who's boss. The cloth of Mary's T-shirt slipped through my fingers. My neck craned behind me. No Mary. Closer to the stage, the emcee's voice boomed, his moist lips pressed the microphone, flecks of spit flew into the crowd. He raised his arm, lifted a flare gun, *POW*!

The momentum carried me onto the course. Mary materialized and flashed me a tight smile.

Wait, so she'd kept me in view the whole time I was freaking out? Was that her idea of a joke?

The crowd thinned as runners and walkers spread out along the course. Mary stuck with me long enough to make sure I was okay, then took off at a dead run looking back over her shoulder just long enough to shout that she'd see me at the finish line.

"You'll lose twenty percent of your lung capacity on the left," said the middle-aged woman in a clipped Indian accent. "But don't worry. You'll never miss it."

Her words settled over me like a shroud.

It was a week after the fun run, and Mary and I were sitting in yet another exam room, this one in Bloomington's unfortunately named Radiation Oncology Center (the ROC for short). Beyond the window, the monotonous gray sky was a reminder that winter was coming and that my active treatment was only half finished.

"We'll try to angle the beam around you heart," said the doctor, "but there are no guarantees. Some collateral damage is inevitable."

For this reason, radiation seemed more insidious than chemo-therapy. The side effects felt more dire. I'd written about how radiation can make the body vulnerable to future cancer diagnoses. How it can destroy cellular DNA, disrupting its ability to divide and multiply. Before cancer, I'd balked when my dentist suggested annual X-rays as a "routine measure." "No thanks," I said brightly, risking being categorized as a fussy patient with trumped up fears about routine medical care—and the label was not far off. But I knew how many X-rays I'd had as a teenager being monitored for scoliosis, and so I didn't take any amount of radiation lightly. With the first diagnosis, side-stepping radiation had weighed into my decision to have a mastectomy. Dr. B had promised that going flat meant no radiation. Now, I had no breasts *and* I was getting radiated. Cancer continued to show me how futile it was to try to control what comes next.

Not only would my risk of radiation-induced cancers be elevated, but if my breast cancer came back on the same side, radiation would no longer be an option, as the same portion of a person's body can only suffer this insult once. And there was something else.

Here's what I'd been too embarrassed to admit: When I chose to go flat, a quiet voice in my head said I could always change my mind later. Reconstruction was still an option. However, once the chest has been radiated, it's no longer a possibility. Or, more accurately, many doctors advise against it because radiated skin no longer stretches or heals as easily as nonradiated skin. It was not until that option disappeared that I realized it had given me peace of mind in case the flat thing didn't work out. I'm someone who likes to keep all of her options open.

A week later we returned to the ROC for "mapping." Mary settled herself by a window with her reading and a cup of vending-machine coffee. A technician took me to a changing room where I took off my shirt and put on a gown. Then she led me deeper inside the building to a darkened room where a half-dozen radiation technicians gathered around me like school kids with an arts and crafts project.

First, she asked me to sit on a metal gurney extending from the mouth of a giant machine like a tongue. Then I was to swing my feet up and extend my legs. Now I'm sitting with my legs in front of me and the business-end of the machine behind me. Someone peels off my hospital gown so I'm naked from the waist up. Now someone puts a large tray of gray slush on the table behind me. Then, two women take hold of my arms and support my weight as I lie back into the tray. Now my back, shoulders, and neck are sinking into the cold, wet mixture, and small, gloved hands are pressing my warm flesh into the frigid ooze.

Had anyone bothered to tell me about the cast? I knew alignment was crucial, thanks to an earlier meeting with Dr. Collateral Damage, but no one had mentioned a cast. Old me would have read up and prepared for such a procedure. Fretted about it. Asked a million questions. But new me had capitulated to the medical establishment. She'd vacated her body, just as you'd move out of a house with cracked walls and a collapsed roof after an earthquake. The plaster firmed its grip on my shoulders and neck as the women darted around the room.

My cast would be labeled with my patient number and hung from clips on a wire that ran along the ceiling. Every radiation patient had one, so that when we arrive at the ROC, a whir of the cables would bring our cast to the front of the line. The system was like the one used by dry cleaners, but instead of freshly laundered pants, blouses, and sweaters whizzing past, the rack held dozens of papier-mâché torsos, waists, and heads—three-dimensional renderings of the town's suffering.

During the hourlong procedure, I kept bracing for the tattoo gun. All the survivors I'd interviewed for articles talked about their tattoos. Some saw the tiny dots as badges of courage, others as painful reminders. Either way, the pinhead-sized dots were a permanent constellation that radiation technicians used to line up the machine. Because they were permanent, the tattoos lowered the risk of human error when positioning the machine's beams.

But instead of a tattoo gun, the technicians at the ROC wielded grease pencils and clear round stickers. The radiation oncologist had given them a list of coordinates corresponding with certain angles. The coordinates were fed into the machine and points of light were projected onto my skin. At each point, the women drew a bright blue "X" an inch high and an inch wide, then covered the mark with a clear sticker. Occasionally the radiation oncologist breezed through the room to check their work.

None of this had been explained to me, at least not in a way that had punctured my chemo-addled brain. And, unsure of what was happening, I stayed quiet. My skin was pale and waxy. My hair was peach fuzz. And my sense of self, the deep knowing of who I was inside my body, had checked out months ago.

By the end, my chest looked like a treasure map. A dozen X's dotted my left side, from my collarbone to my lower rib. Still, I waited for the tattoo gun. Surely that was going to happen any minute.

"Okay, we're finished," a voice said.

Two women grabbed my hands and pulled me up to a sitting position. The cast stayed behind like an exoskeleton.

"What about the tattoos?" I asked in a hoarse whisper.

"What tattoos?"

"You know . . ." I said, my voice faltering. "The tattoos."

"We don't use tattoos," they said.

My heart raced.

"But . . ." I looked down at the grease pencil markings. Clear plastic dots covered the middle of each X but the outer limits of the lines extended beyond the circle's borders. I touched the blue end of an X. It was sticky. The tip of my finger came back blue.

"Just don't touch 'em and you'll be fine," they said.

Don't touch them? My first radiation session was six days away. I'd be getting thirty-six treatments, more than a month's worth.

"But what about showering?" I asked.

"Pat dry," came the response.

Back in the dressing room, I eased into my T-shirt and stopped at the full-length mirror on my way out. Now, in addition to being bald and skeletal, I had several bright blue X's showing above the neckline of my shirt. A few minutes later, in the waiting room, I would finally let my tears go when Mary looked up from her book as I walked toward her. Across her face flashed a sequence of emotions: concern, confusion, and irritation.

"You've got to be kidding me," she said as she got a closer look at my Smurfed skin.

After two major mistakes at the hands of two different doctors, more than anything, I craved reassurance. I needed to trust that my body was being treated with care and precision. No doubt the Smurf-blue X's and their slip-slide stickers were fine. They wouldn't have been used otherwise. But I desperately needed something else, something I didn't have the words to request.

In the days and weeks to come, I was afraid to make a wrong move for fear of disturbing the blue X's. No more washcloths. No more tight-fitting shirts. No more hugs. No more sweating. But, try as I might, one-by-one the protective plastic stickers curled up and slid off, and my faith in the system treating me faded away along with the grease pencil.

"Hey, what time was your radiation again?"

We were at home in our separate offices. Mary had her business voice on. "I need to block that time out on my calendar."

My chest tightened. I'd been meaning to talk with her.

"It's okay. You don't need to go with me." I tried to sound breezy, as if I was just going to the store for salad mix, not the ROC to get my chest fried.

"I know," she said, an edge of impatience creeping into her voice. "I'm planning on driving you every day, but I need to know what time."

"No, really, it's okay," I trilled.

Two seconds later she stood in my office. "What are you saying?"

"Don't be mad, but I think I want to go by myself," I said.

For months Mary had driven me to appointments, arranged for food deliveries, kept track of a half-dozen prescriptions, and even given me post-chemo injections of Neulasta, a drug to boost white blood cell count. I'd surrendered to her care, but now I craved autonomy. To get through thirty-six rounds of radiation, I needed it to be as low-key as possible, just another errand on my daily to-do list. Not an appointment that warranted her accompaniment.

"But this is why I took Family Medical Leave," she shot back. "Remember?" Her face contorted in frustration.

It was true.

Mary had taken a risky move. In the aftermath of my second diagnosis, she'd asked the University for Family Medical Leave, a benefit few of her colleagues dared touch for fear of appearing weak, unable to balance the workload. Her department chair had begrudgingly approved her request and now she was determined to devote herself to my care even more fully than before. It was early September. From the sidelines, she'd been watching her colleagues rev up for fall semester. My reawakening need for independence couldn't have come at a worse time.

"What the hell?" Her arms flew out from her sides, hands up in wide-armed exasperation.

"I'm sorry," I said softly. "I think I just need to do this by myself."

"I can't believe you," she huffed. Then she turned, marched back to her office, and slammed her door.

In anticipation of my needing and wanting her support, Mary had put her job on hold to be present for me, and I wanted nothing more than to be left alone.

A few days later the ritual began.

Five days a week. The alarm clock would buzz. Get up, pull on the same dusty-green pair of sweatpants and a long-sleeve T-shirt. Brush teeth, wash face. Coat, leash, poop bag. Turn to the dog: "Wanna go for a ride?" Brown velvet ears lift. Open the front door, down three concrete steps to the gravel drive, pop open the back of the car. Dog jumps in, circles on her bed, collapses with a humph. Slip behind the wheel and back out of the drive.

Go right at the stop sign. Drive past the neglected bungalows, past the homeless shelter, past the horses grazing in a pasture. At the old gas station, make another right. Go past subdivisions on the right. Woods waiting to be subdivisions on the left. Another stop. Another right. A roundabout. An old quarry. Up the hill. Park at the ROC, same spot across from the front door. Cut the engine. The dog sits up, cocks her head, and watches me walk to the door. Inside the lobby, run my ID through the scanner, like punching a clock at a factory job.

Inside the women's dressing room is a smaller changing area with a door and ten lockers. Off comes my coat, sweater, T-shirt, and jacket. The pumpkin-orange stretchy hat I'd hardly taken off since I lost my hair stays on for warmth. To the right is a folded stack of hospital gowns. Take one off the top, shake it out, slip one arm and then another through the wrinkled sleeves, put the opening in the front, tie the spaghetti ties. Swivel back to face the locker, close the door. Each locker has a key in its lock, and each key is attached to a coiled plastic wristband in a different neon color. I like the bright green one.

Open the door and see a radiation tech waiting. They are alerted to my arrival when I scan my card at the front door. Most likely, my cast has already whooshed down the wire, front of the line. Put on my "good" patient mask, the one belonging to the bright-eyed, chipper cancer patient. Not the morose, depressed, dragging-her-feet-to-the-execution person I am on the inside. "How's your week been?" comes my upbeat question as the tech leads me from the dressing room to the radiation room (aka ground zero). Allowable topics of conversation include: weather, weekend plans, and upcoming holidays. Luckily the trip takes only thirty seconds. As soon as we cross the threshold to the radiation room itself, all small talk ends.

Sit on the metal table. Swing legs up. Lie down. Raise arms overhead. Hold metal handles, one in each hand. Feel shoulders slip into the plaster mold. Two techs on either side peel open the cotton gown and grasp it firmly. With the back of the gown under me, they move my body by tandem tugging the material. Right or left. Up or down. Picture a bedsheet beneath the weight of a body. In that way, I am moved in tiny increments so that the fading blue X's on my torso are aligned in the machine's crosshairs. During this five-minute long nudging, prodding, and pressing, the room is stone-cold silent. If I have to pinpoint a moment when the last crumbs of my identity slip from my grasp, it would be here. Every day. Thirty-six days. A handful of white-clad strangers—both men and women—silently standing over me, tugging my flat, scarred torso into position. My body reduced to a piece of meat. A piece of meat that belongs to them. Them and the disease.

Once happy with my position, the techs admonish me not to move, then slip from the room. The last one out pulls closed a giant lead door. The handle on the outside of the door is a wheel, a foot across and mounted vertically as if on the helm of a ship. I'm afraid to budge, but, if I had, would I have seen it twist and lock, like the door of a submarine? My bare and battered body the only thing in this room not made of steel?

The machine buzzes and whirs to life. Face blinking and clicking. Arms swiveling into preset angles where they stop to deliver a blast of radiation to my chest. I imagine the feeling is akin to being held in the pinchers of a giant nearsighted monster while it peers at you from the left, then the right, to decide how best to devour you.

Zoom up and out of the radiation room. Follow the curve of the road to the east for nearly a mile and you'll see a small parking lot with an access point for the Clear Creek Trail. My salvation. That's why I brought the dog. Every day, after being released from the pinchers, I drive straight to the trailhead, park the car, open the hatchback, and clip Emma's brown leather leash to her collar. The path doesn't look promising at the start. A narrow ribbon of asphalt hemmed in by a twelve-foot chain-link fence on the left and trees on the right. But after a hundred yards or so, the path turns a corner and runs alongside an open field where Emma can run off-leash.

As my feet put distance between me and the car, between me and the machine, everything softens. My face lifts to the weakening September sun. The smell of composting leaves rises from the wet ground. "Go outside and get the stink blown off of you," was my Mother's refrain when we were children. Her voice sticks in my head as the wind presses against the new contours of my body. I picture the wind blowing the radiation off my body, undoing the deep damage to my skin, my tissue, my DNA.

That magical thinking was the only way I was able to return to the ROC every day for thirty-six days.

CHAPTER 23

"We want to see you," my mother said on the phone. "How's this weekend? We could drive up after church."

I hadn't seen my parents in weeks. I knew they were worried but I didn't know how to tell them that I was barely holding it together. That this wasn't a good time for a visit.

During chemo, I'd inched along a tightrope between sadness and depression. Most days I swayed gently between the two, adjusting my footing, easing forward, able to maintain balance and occasionally lift my head to the sky to feel bursts of joy, lightness, and laughter. Talk therapy helped, as did couples therapy. But with the end of chemotherapy, the line went slack and I tumbled.

Everything beyond the scope of my bedroom was overwhelming. Stories needed to be written. Emails begged for replies. Errands went neglected. It took me hours to gather the energy to drive the ten blocks to Bloomingfoods. I'd park facing the door and turn the engine off. I had a list. I had money. I even had a goddamn reusable grocery bag. All I had to do was get out of the car, go into the store, and buy food. But my body refused to move. Hands glued to the steering wheel, I watched as normal-looking people arrived and departed. I was in awe. How did they make it look so easy? Opening the door? Smiling at other shoppers? Making chitchat? I'd slide the key back into the ignition and flick my wrist. As the engine started up, relief flooded through me. The car would spirit me away. Back home, back to the safety of my bed.

Soon, my days looked like this: At 7 a.m., Mary's alarm would go off, she'd roll over, fling an arm in my direction, murmur about wanting just a few more minutes. I'd freeze and pray she didn't open her eyes because my face clearly showed that I'd lain awake since 3 a.m. thinking about death. I took the ten-minute snooze time to rearrange my features into an expression that might pass as calm. Hiding my anxiety-driven inertia from Mary was of utmost importance. She was preparing for our upcoming move to Massachusetts, using every ounce of energy to pull us both up and out of cancer's grasp. When her alarm clock buzzed back to life, I was ready.

We'd get up at 7:20, meaning I only had to act normal for an hour, which was the time Mary would leave the house. In her wake, I'd get up, lash the tie of my blue bathrobe around my waist, straighten the sheets and blankets. My body pleaded with me to turn down the comforter, slip off my robe, and slide between the still-warm sheets, but I assured it that if things went according to plan, that's exactly where I was headed.

In the kitchen I'd make a cup of green tea. Shake organic, flavorless dry cereal into a bowl. Pour rice milk over the top and sit at the table. As Mary ate, I sat in front of my food and watched cardinals and chickadees vie for position at the bird feeder. The birds were eating. Mary was eating—either two poached eggs or toast smeared with a bright yellow pat of melting butter and a tablespoon of peanut butter. Unable to gather the energy to lift my spoon to my lips, I willed the cereal to disappear. As soon as Mary went upstairs to brush her teeth and gather her things, I carried the bowl to the trash can and tipped in the entire soggy mess.

Five minutes later she'd buzz back through the kitchen, plant a kiss on my cheek, and head out the door. The Honda's exhaust pipe sputtered as she pulled away from the curb. I would climb the stairs, walk into the bedroom, and reverse everything we'd just done—close the blinds, pull back the covers on the bed, take off my clothes, and slip between the sheets. I'd lie on my left side, facing the wall. For hours.

I don't remember when I started taking antidepressants or how I even mustered the energy to call the oncologist's nurse and ask for a prescription. By the time my parents decided to drive up to Bloomington for a firsthand look at me, the Lexapro was helping but I was by no means able to hold a normal conversation at a restaurant over brunch. My mother might as well have asked me to fly to the moon.

"Sure," I said. "I'll make a reservation."

And so the next weekend my parents made the two-hour drive from Louisville to Bloomington. I'd made a reservation at a new restaurant near campus called Farm that served fancy comfort food. Unbeknownst to me, it was parents' weekend. When we arrived, the restaurant was overflowing with middle-aged couples and their progeny. The dads wore golf shirts. The moms wore autumnal-themed appliqué cardigans.

We squeezed together at a small table at the front. Around us conversations buzzed, glasses clinked, and silverware clattered. Mary wore her teaching pants, a striped shirt, and her most upbeat face. She flitted between asking my mother about her garden and discussing university politics with my father.

Dressed in a black skirt and a black scoop-necked top, I looked funereal. I was mourning my health; my sense of self; and my inability to protect my body, first from cancer and then from radiation. My parents hadn't seen me bald, but neither mentioned it. Likewise, they didn't call attention to the fact that I was monosyllabic. During the meal I circled round and round their conversation but couldn't find the on-ramp. If it wasn't sports, weather, or family news, I didn't know how to talk with my parents.

My hand reached for Mary's under the table. She held it in her warm grasp, squeezing it every minute or so to let me know she was with me. We'd moved past our fight about driving to radiation, and I imagined my growing independence had given Mary some much-needed breathing room. Cancer had deepened our relationship in ways we didn't fully understand yet. In the past, when Mary's work stress consumed her, I would escape into the familiar fold of my family. Imagine a cliché couple in a sitcom where the wife gets fed up, throws her suitcase in the car, and drives to her mother's house to cool off. That used to be me. But during my two bouts with cancer, Mary was present in a way my family could not be.

Picture me on a raft, drifting out to sea. Sometimes Mary was on the raft. Other times I was alone. Either way, my family stayed on the distant shore. I saw them waving. Smiling. Wanting things on the raft to be okay. They watched as I struggled to stay afloat, but always with a distant, confused look on their faces. Sometimes the raft would drift so far from shore that they would be looking at me with binoculars. Sometimes Mary swam back and forth between the raft and the shore, delivering messages. Sometimes Mary was the raft.

In November, my body continued to disappear. Bundling up in wool sweaters pulled over long-sleeve thermals offered protection from the cold, but my pants drooped and sagged as my waist shrunk and my butt flattened. I rummaged through my closet with my family's annual Thanksgiving trip in mind. Nearing the nadir of my treatment, I'd been in my cancer cocoon for more than six months, not caring what I wore or who saw me. Between my morning trip to the ROC and Clear Creek Trail, I didn't get out much. Every day I pulled on the same pair of sweat pants and tugged the pumpkin-orange knit hat over my fuzzy scalp. But I was going to spend four days with my family, and even though we weren't going anywhere formal, I didn't want to dress the part of a cancer patient.

The next day, I drove to a fancy boutique in downtown Bloomington. The sun was deceptively bright. Crunchy leaves were strewn across roadways and lawns, each bare tree looked mildly surprised at its nakedness. Bells above the door jingled. Two college-aged women behind the counter looked up as if I'd disturbed their private soiree. Before cancer, I would have been too self-conscious to go into an empty store, as being the center of attention was an anathema to me, but cancer had infused me with a what-the-fuck attitude. I hitched up my old jeans, straightened my hat, walked up to the counter, and said that I was finishing breast cancer treatment and that celebratory jeans were in order.

The young women slid off their stools and out from behind the counter to dote on me. They took turns leading me from shelf to shelf to consider stacks of neatly folded denim. They collected styles and cuts for me to try and showed me to the dressing room, a makeshift affair in a corner of the store. Inside, pair after pair of matchstick-thin, Spandex-enhanced denim slipped up over my emaciated thighs. Each zipper came together in front of my hollowed-out gut without protest.

The shopkeepers settled themselves on a purple velvet couch facing the dressing room and purred their approval every time I emerged. With each new pair, one of them would jump up to tug, twist, or torque the fabric. At one point the dark-haired woman sank her thumb into the size-two waistband and yanked, murmuring, "I think you could go down another size." My heart swelled. My body may have been failing at every standard measure of femininity, but for once I was the thinnest woman in the room.

Pathetic. I know. But I was clutching at any perceived fragment of Western womanhood. I'd regressed to adolescent feelings of wanting to be liked and seeking approval from girls who seemed to have cracked the code. In losing my breasts, my curves, and my hair, I'd lost the *femme* in my queer-femme identity. These young women at the jeans shop were willing to overlook my illness and faun over my thinness, and I was only too happy to play along. An hour later, I walked out with a two-hundred-dollar pair of jeans, a steal considering I felt stylish for the first time in two years.

A week later, my family convened at Natural Bridge State Park in central Kentucky. Mary and I were the first to arrive. The afternoon sun was warm and the sky was a thinned wintery-blue.

My family's Thanksgiving tradition was to spend the holiday and the long weekend afterward in one of Kentucky's many state parks. My mom, who loved hiking almost as much as gardening, started the annual trip in 2004 after announcing that, after thirty years of cooking Thanksgiving dinner, she was hanging up her turkey pan. A third generation Kentuckian, my mother has a deep adoration of the state. Not interested in camping, especially in the winter, my mom picked a different state park each year, one with a lodge, restaurant, and cabins. My parents and me and Mary stayed in lodge rooms, while my three siblings and their growing families got cabins for the duration. Every morning we'd fill our bellies with watery scrambled eggs, greasy hash browns, and waffle sticks swimming in syrup—this was rural Kentucky after all, and the food is not all that—and every afternoon and most evenings we'd converge in a cabin to cook and play games. My mother was relaxed and happy, which made all of us relaxed and happy. The new Thanksgiving tradition quickly became my favorite holiday. I wasn't about to miss it, and this year it had extra significance as the Thanksgiving that marked the end of radiation. My body could finally rest and heal.

"Let's go for a hike," Mary said. She grinned. The braided ends of her Pippi Longstocking hat bouncing with excitement.

I looked at the trailhead leading up to the park's famous Natural Bridge.

"It looks steep."

"You can do it. We'll go slow."

My body was thin but I wasn't as weak or wobbly as I had been during chemo. The trail was less than a mile, and, according to the map, there were benches along the way. I tugged the sides of my orange knit hat down over my ears. "Okay, if we are going to get back before dinner, we should get going."

We started up the trail. I'd expected my legs to feel rubbery and weak but instead my muscles responded to the gentle uphill grade as if waking up from a long nap. As we climbed through the forest of white pine and hemlocks, my body warmed and my face flushed. When I got winded, which was often, we'd stop and rest. Slowly, we made our way up the trail. I took huge gulps of air. Grateful to be outside. Grateful that my body felt capable. And, after so many solo walks after radiation, grateful to be doing this together. For the first time in a long time, I was at Mary's side and I was not slowing her down. When we got to the top of the limestone bridge, we stopped to gaze out over the treetops, the rolling hills, the rocky outcroppings. How far we'd come.

Mary pulled me to her, wrapping her arms around my shoulders, my hands naturally clasped behind her waist. I nestled my face into the crook of her neck and felt the strength of her body as well as the calm, confident optimism at her core.

That weekend, Mary and I went on more short hikes, played charades, goofed off with our nieces and nephews. I wore my new jeans every day. My parents and siblings each let me know in their own way, with an extra-long hug here or a squeeze there, that they loved me and were trying to respect my request that we discuss cancer only if I was the one who brought it up. Mary and I had worked out a system where she made herself available for their questions and I let them know I was fine with them discussing my health with her. Everyone had as much information as they wanted, but I didn't have to rehash the ins and outs of chemotherapy and radiation with each person. And, several times over the long weekend, I glimpsed Mary hanging back on hikes with one of my sisters or grabbing a ride to town with my mom to create some one-on-one time to answer questions. My heart filled seeing how much my family members loved and trusted Mary. How safe they felt confiding in her. That weekend, for the first time, it became clear to me that my relationship with Mary nurtured and enhanced my relationship with my family. I didn't need to choose one over the other.

CHAPTER 24

On January 2, 2011, we put Emma in the car and drove to New England. Somerville was a dense New England town pressed up against Cambridge. If Greater Boston were a family, Cambridge would be the first-born overachiever, an intellectual striver, and a people pleaser. Somerville would be the middle child, funky, laid-back, and always up for a party. As a middle child myself, Somerville suited me just fine.

In Inman Square the houses were packed like teeth, rooflines jostled for space, and lawns were the size of doormats. Our street was tucked behind a two-block business district with a coffee shop, a hardware store, a post office, and Christina's Ice Cream. All of my needs were met within a five-minute walk. Our home for six-months was a small apartment buried in the belly of an older house. The owners, a dog-loving lesbian couple, lived upstairs. The apartment was a bit dark, but it was warm and cozy, and it was ours. I felt enclosed and protected. No more big-eyed windows staring out at the four-way intersection. No more bus stop, fistfights, and fender benders. No more living room with two doors opening straight to the outside world. This was a comfortable, quiet place to heal.

Before leaving Indiana, I'd had one last meeting with Dr. Muppet. He asked if I'd gotten my period. Nope. I hadn't bled since the girls' weekend at Lake Michigan six months prior. He looked pleased. With my ovaries offline, my odds of yet another cancer scare were lower. Talk of hormone therapy was on hold for now. We were all hoping my period's six-month hiatus would translate into early-onset menopause. But, just in case, he wrote down the name of an oncologist in Boston. I tucked the paper into the accordion file where I kept my health records, and Mary and I floated out of his office on the hope that we'd never see him or the Simon Cancer Center again.

In hindsight, I probably misinterpreted his farewell as goodbye for good and not just for the six months Mary and I would be on the East Coast. I was so eager to escape. To enter a witness protection program for cancer patients. According to my magical thinking, as long as my body was in menopause, I was home free.

Within days I fell in love with my new city. In part because no one in Somerville or Cambridge knew I'd had cancer. If I wanted someone to know, I could choose to share my history, but it was a choice, not universal knowledge. For the first time in two years, my former identity as a healthy person was within reach.

In Bloomington, whether I was at the food co-op, the yoga studio, or my favorite coffee shop, people would ask about my cancer. One minute we'd be talking about the weather, an upcoming yoga workshop, or holiday plans, and the next minute the friend would lower their voice and ask, "So. Really. How *are* you?" Once you've inhabited the world of the sick, you no longer travel unencumbered through the world of the healthy.

In Cambridge, on my first foray to the Trader Joe's near Fresh Pond, my phone rang; it was Beth.

"You sound so happy," she chuckled.

"That's because I'm in the middle of a crowded grocery store and I don't know a single person!"

I danced a jig in the frozen food aisle.

"Sheesh, you're such a nerd."

Inside the one-bedroom apartment, I carved out a small work space with a diminutive desk. Determined to pick up the pieces of my career, I made a list of editors to pitch to and tried to stay upbeat about my prospects as a magazine freelancer, knowing the industry had gone through an upheaval while I was in treatment.

The burgeoning world of online content combined with the 2008 recession had delivered a series of blows to print publishing. Many of the smaller women's magazines had shuttered and even the larger ones were on life support. Everyone was reorganizing and cutting staff. My phone began to ring. Editors were calling, but not with assignments. They'd been laid off and were asking me the same questions: How do you freelance? What accounting software do you use? What's the best way to track pitches? Who's buying?

Soon, we were all competing against one another for a shrinking number of assignments. Bloating our ranks were hundreds of daily news journalists cut loose from the nation's starving newspapers. We were all scrambling for paid work. Websites had an unquenchable thirst for content, but few felt the need to pay writers a livable wage. Print magazines had paid one to two dollars a word, enough to squeak out a living. Now web clients were offering pennies a word for similar assignments.

My goal for our six months in Somerville/Cambridge was to scrape together part-time magazine work and to walk the dog. The dog was deliriously happy with this arrangement and Mary, with her fellowship more than paying the bills, gave me her blessing. At the start, that's what I did. Emma was ten years old and spritely. We'd exposed her to city life as a puppy and now she was unfazed by police sirens, crowded sidewalks, and honking cars. Mary, ever the studious one, had invested countless hours in leash training Emma early on and I continued to reap the rewards of a well-trained dog. Emma trotted at my side, just close enough to leave slack in the leash. She pulled up at intersections, gathering her haunches under her as if to sit, but really coiling into a spring. At my command she'd push off into a trot. She was curious and confident, easy-going and energetic. She seemed happiest, ears relaxed, gait perky, when we were exploring new territory, and Cambridge held such dog-walking treasures as the campuses of Harvard and MIT and the band of green parkland running along the Charles River.

Emma and I spent the first two weeks exploring the streets of Somerville and Cambridge. My only ambition: not to travel the same sidewalk twice. We moseyed up and down cobblestone sidewalks that rose and fell like rollercoasters thanks to pushy tree roots. Tiny green spaces materialized every few blocks, perfectly kept. And, maybe it was my early attachment to the Peterson Palace, but my heart swelled at the sight of the city's architecture. Secret gardens, hidden doorways, attic apartments with dormer windows that glowed like warm hearts. Blocks upon blocks of hundred-plus-year-old homes, some lovingly restored, some falling apart. Most were carved into a curious number of apartments. Many hid carriage houses and even the occasional barn behind their wide girths. Not since San Francisco had I lived in a place so architecturally rich. The tenacity and creativity of the cities' inhabitants was inspiring. People's capacity for carving out space for themselves, for creating new worlds.

For the first time since my cancer diagnosis, I was excited to get out of bed in the morning. Living in Somerville sparked my imagination, made me consider what life I might create with my second chance. I would like to say that my story ends on this upbeat note. That Mary, Emma, and I lived happily ever after. That, as my oncologist liked to say, "Cancer was in my review mirror." But that's not exactly how things unfolded.

Within the month, Mary had to travel to New York on business. I drove her to Logan Airport. We dawdled at the departures drop-off, engine idling, hazard lights ticking. Inside the car, our breath fogged the windshield as a stream of taxis, SUVs, and minivans popped people and bags out on the curb. My gloved fingers curled and uncurled around the steering wheel. Mary fumbled with her phone, her gloves, her hat.

Beneath her down jacket she wore a heather-brown sweater over a button-down shirt with stripes. Two dozen striped shirts in various hues hung in tight formation on identical wood hangers in the closet of our new apartment. The predictability of her wardrobe, like that of her world, taunted me. That and her ambition. Mary was going places.

"You know I have to go, right? Everybody at work is going."

"Yeah, I know."

She kissed me and slipped out of the car, pausing on the sidewalk to thread her arms through the straps of her backpack. The car shimmied as the door slammed. She tossed me a wave and hurried through the sliding glass doors of the terminal. That was Mary—always hurrying, always focused on the next thing. Seeing her hustle through the sliding glass doors reminded me of the evening twelve years ago when I'd followed her red raincoat down Valencia Street. Now, she'd been invited to join researchers at one of the world's largest tech companies. This was a chance for Mary to turn her energy back to her career, to recharge and refocus. She needed a cancer vacation as much as I did. Even getting tenure at Indiana University—what should have been the highlight of her young career—had been overshadowed by my cancer.

"Ooouuw." Emma yawned from the back of the car. She stretched her long neck, the white blaze on her chest flashed, her fawn muzzle brushing the ceiling. Resetting my GPS for an errand south of the city, I steered the car out of the airport and onto I-93. Twenty minutes later, back on surface streets, my eyes searched for a place to exercise the dog, somewhere she could run off-leash.

Since our early-January arrival, more than sixty inches of snow had fallen on the city. The absence of yards and space between houses created a mind-boggling logistical challenge—the new snow had to be shoveled off sidewalks and drives, but there was no place to put it. Sidewalks became gullies of ice between steep walls of snow. I'd been on the prowl for off-leash green spaces were Emma could run off her ya yas.

There, up ahead—a field, trees, a trail. I pulled the Subaru over into what looked like a makeshift parking lot and popped the hatchback. Emma leapt from the car like a frog from a Mason jar. Snort. Wiggle. Shake. She bounded across the snow as if to taunt me with her spry grace. My progress was slower.

Ice crackled underfoot. The midday sun glared off the snow. Every few yards, without warning—*ka-wamp!*—the ground disappeared. Crunch, crunch, *ka-wamp*! Crunch, crunch, *ka-wamp*! As my boot broke the surface, my weight was thrown forward and down. Rolling snowstorms had dumped six to ten inches at a time. Between each blizzard was a blue-sky day, the sun enough to melt the top layer of snow into an icing-like glaze. Each night the layer froze anew.

Across the field, Emma's barks shattered the air above the woodsy mouth of a trail. From the road the field had appeared a simple white space. A blank sheet upon which a big dog might scribble herself silly. But she'd traced no scribbles, no loopy figure eights. She'd drawn a straight line from the car to the field's border and a shaggy opening in a wall of evergreens. Overhead, a seagull swung in slow circles. My lungs exchanged the crisp, empty air for the lingering chaos of Logan Airport.

By the time I seriously considered turning around the trees were closer than the car.

Why had this seemed like a good idea?

Why hadn't I simply steered toward home?

My stomach queased. The snow refused to offer any clues of instability—no indentations or shadows to suggest a weakness. Sweat broke out under my arms. My wool scarf, prickly and damp, had a stranglehold on my neck.

Zoom out and back a year to the night Mary had unfolded a map of Boston across my lap. I'd been drawn to the blue ribbon of the Charles River, the crosshatching of unfamiliar streets, red stripes denoting the boundaries of Boston, Cambridge, and Somerville. A flutter stirred in my chest. A younger version of myself had moved sight unseen to

Denver and, later, San Francisco. But, post-cancer, I'd considered my days of picking up and starting over finished.

Now fast-forward a year, drag your eyes back to the Northeast. That dot in the snowfield was me. Zoom in closer and you would have heard Emma barking. Look closer still and you might have seen that something about me was not right. My face was a young woman's, but my body was that of an old man. My hair was patchy and Brillo-pad short, my muscles withered, my left arm out of sorts. Thirty-six rounds of radiation had melted the muscles of my upper arm into a congealed mass, hard like the plastic beads in the Shrinky Dinks kits my siblings and I played with as kids.

Layers of snow and ice snapped beneath my feet. Emma bound ahead, stopping only once to twist her thick boxer neck around to look at me and offer an encouraging bark. Finally, my feet found solid ground at the far edge of the snow field, under a canopy of eastern white pines. Emma and I were alone with the sharp scent of pine needles, chatter of nuthatches, and occasional *ffffomp* of snow sliding off a tree branch.

The dog zigzagged down the nearby path, tracing a scent, so I eased into a relaxed stride and followed along. After a quarter of a mile, a wisp of a trail led down a hill. The crumbled leaves hinted at foot traffic. Curious as to what drew locals from their cozy, lamp-lit homes into the frozen woods in January, I picked my way down the narrow thread. At the bottom of the hill, a clearing revealed a skating pond, hardly bigger than a backyard pool.

I'd only read about things like skating ponds in the pages of Hans Christian Andersen. A closer look revealed simple wooden benches bookending the ice. Snowflakes on the ice looked like confetti after a party. The ice's surface held the traces of lines, circles, and figure eights like a well-used Etch A Sketch. The movement of the lines were so energetic I could almost see the pink cheeks, hear the shouts, smell the hot chocolate.

But the sun was setting. It was time to go. I whistled for the dog and retraced my steps. The snowfield was waiting, and this time my footprints would show me the way out.

First things first, I needed to pee.

I squatted behind a tree, inched my jeans toward my knees, then stood up, zipped my pants, and started to scuff snow over the yellow patch. But the snow wasn't yellow. It was red. Bright red. My period had started. A distant tree branch cracked under the weight of its burden.

A sob stuck in my throat. The blood wept into the snow. The dog whined a skinny complaint. A plane hummed overhead.

My heart pounded. My eyelids clamped shut, willing the scene to start over. But when I opened them it was still there . . . proof that my ovaries were back online. I wanted to curse my uncooperative body. To lie down and yell uncle at the trees, at the sky, at the universe. Blood meant estrogen, and estrogen was my cancer's jet fuel.

Why wouldn't my body capitulate? Give in to the chemotherapy that had shocked my ovaries into shutting down last summer? I wanted to be done with doctors, hospitals, and illness, but here in the woods, in a city, state, and region where I knew no one, where I'd come to escape cancer's shadow, my ovaries had sputtered back to life. For the first time, I was mad at my body.

Would my body's resilience be my undoing?

Forget the fifteen hundred miles I'd put between myself and the Simon Cancer Center, Dr. B and the mistakes. Forget the imaginary longitudinal line I'd drawn on the map to divide my pre-and post-cancer life. Forget my fantasy of a cancer-free existence in Somerville. The precious time I'd set aside to reboot my writing career would be shot through with doctors' appointments, tests, and procedures. The witness protection program had failed me.

Back in the car I yanked off my gloves, blasted the heat, and dug deep into my coat pocket for my phone. I pressed the cold metal rectangle to my ear and heard Mary's voicemail chirp. I hung up, pictured the way my name and the words "missed call" would pop up on the screen of her phone when she landed at LaGuardia, and thought of Mary trying to get on with her life and me yanking her back into the world of cancer.

At the apartment I rooted through boxes looking for the slip of paper the Muppet had handed me two months before, the same day Mary and I had all but skipped out of his office, buoyed by the hope that I was in early menopause.

On the bottom shelf of the bookcase was the brown accordion file, the one that held my thick stack of health records, the same file I'd hoped not to need again but was too paranoid to leave behind at our house in Indiana. On a sheet of paper was the name of a Boston oncologist. Someone I'd hoped to never meet. And I wouldn't, at least not today. It was Sunday, and the light in the room was fading. Fuzzy snores rose from Emma's dog bed as my palm smoothed the wrinkled paper flat on the surface of the writing desk.

CHAPTER 25

On the day of my first oncology appointment in Boston, a freak February rainstorm soaked the city. Melting snow flooded the streets. When the bus deposited me and Mary on the sidewalk in front of the Dana-Farber Cancer Institute, we were drenched. The glass doors parted, our rain boots squeaked on the polished floor, and my stomach somersaulted.

I'd followed research emanating from Harvard University and its affiliated cancer research arm Dana-Farber the way more normal people might follow their favorite authors or musicians. I'd poured over the Harvard Medical School's publications looking for story ideas, health trends, and new sources to interview. In my home office back in Bloomington, Harvard Health Publications were neatly arranged in three-ring binders—a binder for each year—and given a place of prominence on my bookshelf. I'd always imagined I would visit the Dana-Farber Cancer Institute one day on a press junket. I never imagined I'd walk through the door as a patient.

The elevator rose to the breast cancer center on the ninth floor. We stepped out into a reception area decorated in shades of blue, green, and gray. Floor-to-ceiling windows looked out on the surrounding city scape. Through the rain-streaked glass, the midrise buildings looked as winter-weary as I felt. Dana-Faber was home to my new oncologist, Dr. P, a Harvard-trained MD, MPH, who specialized in treating young breast cancer patients. Mary and I took two seats near a window. She took my hand, her warm fingers wrapping around my cool palm.

At her tech-company job across the Charles, Mary worked as hard as ever, yet this morning she didn't pull out a book or reach for her phone to fire off a quick email. She sat with me in my misery. No attempts to fix things were made. Whereas before we would have pulled into the safety of our shells, now we stuck around for one another.

After a short wait, we were taken back to yet another beige exam room, and after a few more minutes, in walked a tall woman with shoulder-length curly, red hair and shimmering blue eyes. She was around my age, a welcome change from patrician men. She extended her hand to me and Mary and flashed us a wide smile. "I hear Dr. S sent you to me. He's one of the best." She did a quick introduction and gave us a short overview of what was going to happen during the visit. First, a brief exam. She palpated the lymph nodes in my neck and under my arms, her hands confident and firm. Afterward, she put down my file, sat down on the desk chair, and crossed her legs.

"So, I've spent some time with your chart." She paused, popping her eyebrows and tucking her chin. In my imagination, I saw her flipping through the dozens of pages detailing my experience at Simon Cancer Center in Indianapolis, including the mistake, the second mastectomy, and the lentil surprise. "I can imagine you've lost a bit of faith in the medical system." I nodded. My shoulders softened at her lack of pretense, her acknowledgement that mistakes chip away at patient confidence.

Without a clipboard, a laptop, or any other props between us, there was a sense of two people staring at a formidable problem. She exuded confidence without condescension. Leaning back in her chair, she swept a curl away from her forehead and looked me in the eye. "What we need is a new plan." Her let's-figure-this-out-together tone caught me off guard. Doctors typically had strong opinions about what I should do next. "Normally, I'd have some statistics to help guide your decision, but, honestly, your case is so outside the norm that the statistics no longer apply to you. You're in a data-free zone."

Her observation was so honest, so human.

"So, tell me, what's important to you?" she asked, her eyes meeting mine. "Are you an 'exhaust all treatment options, no matter how crappy they make you feel' kinda person? Or are you a person who would rather live with a little more uncertainty, meaning less treatment, if it meant you felt better day-to-day?"

No doctor had ever asked me about my preference. I was not a risk-taker by nature, but if something seemed reasonable, I was willing to try it. However, if the side effects made me miserable, I wasn't willing to sacrifice years of my life to a drug therapy that may or may not work. I told her this.

She nodded and said, "This is your life. You've gotta enjoy it."

We decided to try the standard therapy and check back in a few months.

For my estrogen-sensitive breast cancer, standard therapy meant hormone suppression. Tamoxifen, which had failed me, is the first line of defense. The second option for pre-menopausal women was a combination of two drugs—Lupron plus an aromatase inhibitor. Lupron stops the pituitary gland from making luteinizing hormone, a biochemical that goads the ovaries into releasing estrogen. Lupron's sidekick is the aromatase inhibitor (AI for short), designed to squeegee out the estrogen made outside the ovaries, primarily fat tissue. AIs work by stopping an enzyme in fat tissue, called aromatase, from changing other hormones into estrogen.

In the following weeks, I swallowed a daily AI and got a monthly Lupron shot. Common side effects of both Lupron and AIs were joint pain, night sweats, moodiness, and brain fog. Although I had all of the above, the most frustrating side effect was fatigue. My energy plummeted. No more meandering dog walks to the Longfellow House in Cambridge or on Somerville's Minuteman Trail. My days were spent moving from the bed to the writing desk and back to bed again.

Mary encouraged me to keep a journal of my symptoms, something to take to my next appointment with Dr. P. Something concrete that would show the impact of the drugs over time. Looking back on that notebook makes me wince:

tired
nap
cranky/sad
hot flashes
major tooth grinding
cry easily

Losing my body's estrogen was, in many ways, more difficult than losing my breasts. Changes to the outside of my body—the way the world saw me and how I negotiated my body in space and in relationship to others—were difficult but manageable. But losing my sense of who I was on the inside was deeply unsettling.

To distract myself from my new "inside problem," I sought healing for my "outside problems." Radiation had thickened and hardened the layers of muscle in my upper left arm. Normally the layers would glide over one another like fish in a barrel. Now things felt stuck. Small movements, like putting on a seat belt in the car or reaching back to put my arm in a coat sleeve, were challenging.

So, twice a week I put Emma in the car and drove to Cindy's office in a distant western suburb of Boston—an hour each way with traffic and often in snow—in hopes she could help me regain full range of motion. Unlike the physical therapist my parents had taken me to for my scoliosis, Cindy specialized in gentle techniques, such as craniosacral therapy, visceral manipulation, and myofascial release. Gradually, as winter turned to spring, she separated the fused layers of fascia, muscle, and tendons in my shoulder. Her techniques might have been considered a bit woo-woo among conventional physical therapists, but there was nothing hippy-dippy about her. She wore business attire and a white lab coat. She had a thriving practice, employing several other physical therapists. When I showed up for an appointment, a receptionist led me into a tastefully decorated treatment room that contained a massage-style table. Like all the patients, I changed into a hospital gown that tied in the back.

But there was an element to these visits that I hadn't foreseen. Cindy worked skin-on-skin. Her hands on my bare chest. Sometimes she used just her fingertips to release scar tissue around my incisions. Other times she'd knead the deep muscles of my chest and shoulder using the flat palm of her hand and push, press, and mold my body. My guess is that my chest appeared to be a desexualized swath of skin and bone. But my brain hadn't gotten the message. Whenever she touched the area where my breasts had been, my brain sounded an alarm. Stranger in the breast zone! It was all I could do not to leap off the table.

I should have said something, but I feared it would make her more hesitant to deliver the therapy that was helping me recover my mobility. After a session with Cindy, my shoulder felt more spacious, my arm moved more freely, and the curve in my upper back felt better than it had in years. Cindy never brought up the fact that she was massaging my bare chest. And why would she? She wasn't thinking about my breasts. She'd never seen me with breasts. I wondered if, in her eyes, my chest looked like a man's. Would she have asked a male patient for permission to touch his chest? Occupying a body that, for some, could fall into this gray area was odd but also strangely normal. This was me now. Just as I'd eventually stopped feeling self-conscious about coming out to people as queer. I lived my life, talked about my partner, and never made accommodations for other people's discomfort. If they had feels, they could work them out. Similarly, my flat-chested body was simply a part of who I was now. No excuses necessary.

Living close to Dana-Farber also gave me access to workshops and support I never could have gotten in Bloomington. In March, I signed Mary and me up for a workshop called "Sex After Breast Cancer." A psychologist led the discussion, describing the toll surgeries and hormone therapies take on a couple's intimacy.

But it wasn't until the end of the presentation that she said the words I needed to hear: "It's okay not to like the way you look after cancer. It's okay not to like your body. If you don't like what you see, cover it up." My ears buzzed. I glanced around the room. What? What was that? Did she just give me permission to *not* like my body?

It was all I could do to keep from jumping out of my folding chair and kissing the workshop facilitator. Mary raised an eyebrow as if to say, "Is this really what you are taking away from this class?" But I smiled and sat back in my seat as something deep inside of me softened.

I'd been thinking in terms that were way too black-and-white. I had loved my body once, but I was struggling to love the version of myself that didn't have breasts. Somehow I'd forgotten that I still had plenty of other parts of my body that hadn't changed. I still loved my muscular legs, the curve of my upper arms, and the strength in my hands. When Mary and I had sex, there was plenty of pleasure to be had from her tongue, hands, and fingers working their magic between my legs. I gave myself permission that day to cover my scars in bed.

CHAPTER 26

In early August, Mary and I packed up our little Somerville apartment and drove back to Bloomington. Our six-month adventure was finished. Deep down, a part of me hoped we'd pick up our lives where we'd left off before cancer. I'd slip back into the groove of writing at the white desk, pulling weeds along the picket-fence, and teaching yoga on Wednesday nights. Mary would return to teaching and publishing but without the high-pressure stakes of tenure. We'd get back into the habit of long evening dog walks and weekend trips to the Peterson Palace.

And, at first, things looked promising. A tornado that had touched down in our neighborhood while we were gone had spared our house and Lorraine's across the street. And we were relieved to see that Pearl, the flowering pear tree we'd planted in the front yard to replace the towering water maple, was still standing. We could not say the same for the sagging, white-picket fence so we had a new one built, and I had grand plans for painting it. I was already lining up next summer's outdoor projects. Our twelfth dating anniversary was in early August, and we celebrated by walking downtown to the Indiana Theatre, the town's Art Deco theater, to see *Breaking Away*, the only Hollywood movie ever filmed in Bloomington. We bought crinkly bags of salty popcorn, sat in the back row, elbowed each other, and pointed at recognizable streets and buildings. On the way home, we held hands, choosing smaller, moonlit streets over the busier thoroughfares. Our bodies relaxed into the ease of small town life.

But, in the coming weeks, the side effects of my hormone suppressants hit an unbearable new level. I'll never know if it was the heat and humidity of the midwest or if the medication was reaching maximum potency in my body, but each monthly Lupron injection left me swimming through my days, unable to concentrate, much less articulate about what was happening. The inability to focus made reading and comprehension difficult, which made reporting nearly impossible. My brain no longer recognized rhythm in writing or music. I couldn't read my own writing aloud to hear if the edges of the words fit smoothly or rubbed awkwardly. Even the playlists Mary had burned for me, the soundtrack to every car ride, sounded flat and hard.

There were changes to my body, too. Hot flashes pulsed through me a dozen times a day. A rush of deep-furnace heat that left me peeling off layers. My joints swelled and ached. After sitting, I struggled to stand, unable to straighten my knees or my hips. At night, while I slept, the tendons of my fingers tightened until my hands turned into claws. Every morning I had to pry my fingers open, one at a time, before getting out of bed. During the day, my swollen, stiff finger joints meant I couldn't hold a pen or grip the car's steering wheel. Unable to pull weeds, we hired a gardener for the yard. Unable to walk more than a few dozen feet, Mary took Emma to Bryan Park by herself. I took ibuprofen. I tried acupuncture and meditation. I ate an anti-inflammatory diet. Nothing helped.

My follow-up care had transferred back to Dr. Muppet, but my calls to his office went unreturned. After a couple of rambling voice mail messages during which I described my symptoms in detail and begged him to see me, his nurse called back, "We've never heard of joint pain being a side effect of hormone therapy. You must have developed osteoarthritis."

"But my joint pain started a few weeks after I started the drug protocol. Arthritis progresses in years, not months."

"Do you want a referral to a rheumatologist?" she asked, her voice brisk.

"But rheumatologists aren't trained in breast cancer hormone therapies, they won't know what to do with me."

"I'm sorry," she said. "That's the best we can do."

Teaching yoga was a torment. During weeks lost to Lupron-brain, remembering the Sanskrit names of poses, much less the sequences, was impossible. The cues for each pose that normally ticked through my head had vaporized. The melodic playlist I'd made to set the mood sounded like pans clattering in the background. After weeks of struggling, Mary came to support me, her purple mat stretched out in the front row. I fought my way through class with my creaky body and useless brain. On the way home, tears streamed down my face. Out came weeks of frustration and sadness at what my brain and body could no longer do. As she drove, she struggled to calm my fears, telling me that no one had noticed, that the class went off without a hitch. But instead of feeling reassured, I felt invisible. The next day I told Lucy I couldn't do it anymore, and that was it. I'd taught my last yoga class. Side effects from the estrogen-blockers had commandeered every corner of my life.

Being inside the milk-carton house felt as uncomfortable as being inside my body. Memories of cancer haunted me. The bedroom where the lump had revealed itself, the white whale of a desk where two callers—eighteen months apart—had told me I had cancer, even the brown couch. That damn brown couch held every body memory of chemotherapy—the nausea, the penetrating bone aches, the skin-crawling fidgets. Soon after we moved back into the house, Emma got violently ill on the lily pad of a braided wool rug we'd had in the living room. When every cleaning solution tried and failed to erase the smell, we rolled it up and put it on the curb. The bare hardwood floors made the living room bright and clean, and, with the pads under the feet of the brown couch, I began to push it around the room in hopes that a new configuration would cleanse my palette of its chemotherapy aftertaste. The brown couch had two sections, which opened up my options considerably. Every day it found its way into a different arrangement and location in the room.

Upstairs things were more static. Wall-to-wall carpeting on my office floor and the size of my desk kept me from moving the furniture, but in hindsight, maybe that's what my career needed. Magazine work was drying up. When assignments came, the Lupron made it difficult for me to multitask. Whereas I'd once juggled half a dozen different stories at a time—jumping from topic to topic, researching and inter-viewing—now my brain could focus on just one topic at a time. Less able to think on my feet, my interviews required more preparation. And writing took twice as long because organizing my thoughts into a logical sequence took hours. I chose assignments with more care, limiting myself to working with known editors, people who would understand if I needed a deadline extension.

Just as the cancer had dislodged my identity as a healthy person and the double mastectomy had undone my sense of femininity, Lupron was threatening my ability to write, usurping my sense of self.

When a young editor from *Better Homes and Gardens* called and dangled a five-thousand-dollar assignment—a roundup of the year's top advances in breast cancer—my gut said, "Don't do it." The Seven Sisters, of which *Better Homes and Gardens* belonged to, was a group of women's magazines that, during their heyday, had a combined circula-tion of 45 million readers. Their editors had a wicked reputation for being impossible to please. Professional freelancers I met online and at conferences told horror stories about endless rounds of revisions, inaccuracies inserted into articles, and editors killing stories at the last minute. But one look at my bank account put my doubts in the backseat.

In the early days of negotiating the terms of the contract, my rela-tionship with the young editor blossomed like a romance. We exchanged witty email banter. She was honest and forthcoming about the maga-zine's terrible reputation among writers, but even as she empathized with me, she assured me this time would be different. She promised to protect me from endless revisions and last-minute rewrites. Then she went one step further and got approval from her top editors to move forward with the piece, saving me from writing a lengthy, time-consuming proposal. Writers aren't paid for writing proposals, and many times the idea is shot down at the proposal stage, which leaves the writer with nothing to show for her work. So, after nailing down a detailed outline, I signed the contract and got to work.

For the next six weeks, I worked on the story through my Lupron haze. My initial fears of a dearth of new science were unfounded. Although true groundbreaking advances in breast cancer prevention, drugs, and treatments were few and far between, progress had been made that year: the FDA approved 3-D mammograms, which were thought to have an advantage over the traditional format. New surgical protocols changed the way lymph nodes were removed, meaning fewer side effects and lower odds of lymphedema. Other solid advances rounded out the piece. My choices were backed up with new peer-reviewed research and more than two dozen interviews with the top breast cancer researchers in the country.

I wrote, rewrote, and revised the story. I was proud of the piece. Between jacking myself up on coffee and then allowing myself to nap when I crashed, I'd kept my mind focused on the research and writing.

Two days after filing the story, the young editor called.

"Um, this story isn't working for me."

"Really, why?"

"The science is just so . . . science-y," she said. "You're not speaking to our demographic."

"Women?"

"Our readers are ladies sitting on their expensive sofas in West-chester, New York. They want to be entertained, not read about research." Gone was the witty banter, the assurances of teamwork. Her voice was ice.

I stammered about the outlines I'd sent her, the abstracts, the source list she'd approved.

"Yeah, well, I don't like it. You need to rewrite it," she said. "I have some ideas that might work."

She went on to tell me about a hospital in Chicago offering women free manicures with their mammograms. "Isn't that a great idea! Now *that* is what I want to see in this story!"

I don't remember what I said but I managed to get off the phone before I lost my shit. The next day I spent way too much energy writing a thoughtful explanation of why the science was important.

The young editor replied that a hundred freelance writers would be happy to take the job if I wasn't willing to write about free manicures as a breakthrough in women's health.

In the nicest way I knew how, I asked her to reconsider. She fired me.

I'm saying all this because this was the point at which I understood that cancer had forever changed the way I approached my job as a women's health journalist. After years of following editors orders to sugarcoat breast cancer stories, I couldn't do it anymore. I felt a moral obligation to not only take the topic seriously but to also tell women the full story. If that made me a less-desirable magazine journalist, then so be it.

Two months later, Mary was offered a full-time position at the tech company's research lab in Cambridge. The job meant stepping away from her post as a tenured professor, the very thing she'd worked so hard to achieve. But she knew I missed Massachusetts. She'd been watching me struggle to find the equilibrium I'd lost since moving back to Indiana. Every day when she came home from work, the brown couch was in a different corner of the living room and I was in bed under the covers. She accepted the job. First, she would finish out the academic year in Bloomington. That would be just enough time for us to sell our white rectangle house with its black eyeliner and ruby-red mouth.

In 2012, we moved to Somerville and set about making a new home. I spent the first eighteen months trying different drug combinations of adjuvant hormone therapy in hopes of finding a magic formula that would wipe out my estrogen without destroying my quality of life. I never found it. And, the following year, with the full support of Dr. P, my fierce, fiery Boston oncologist, I went off hormone therapy altogether.

I've taken a risk in going off the medication meant to suppress my body's estrogen production. Both of my breast cancer tumors were estrogen-receptor positive, so there is a chance my unchecked estrogen could spark a new growth or even fuel metastatic disease. No doubt, some people will see this choice as irresponsible. But here are some things that seem to help the body keep cancer at bay: solid sleep, lots of exercise, and (possibly) lowering inflammation. None of those things were possible for me while I was on the hormone-lowering drug. So I made a choice to follow the same gut-instinct that led me to go flat—I went with what felt best for my body.

I'd be remiss if I didn't say that a lack of data also played into my decision. So little information matched my situation—a woman in her thirties with two primary tumors, both estrogen-positive, and at least one that grew on Tamoxifen. As my oncologist and I whittled down my options, she reiterated that I was "in a data-free zone." There were no guarantees that hormone therapy would benefit me. It's dangerous to play the "what if" game, but if doctors could offer me reasonable assurances that a drug would keep recurrence at bay, I can imagine I'd take it in a heartbeat. But no one had any statistics that matched my situation, meaning my reasons for staying on the drugs were increasingly weighted toward fear. Fear that the cancer would come back and kill me. Fear of more pain and suffering. Eventually, fear was ruling my life, which felt all too familiar. I'd grown up fearing my body. In high school, I feared my fused spine. In college, my fear of being friendless led me to join a sorority. Not until I befriended my body and came fully out of the closet in San Francisco did I overcome my fear. Coincidentally or not, when I stopped living in fear, I met Mary. Later, my confidence allowed me to tune into my body deeply, a skill that ultimately allowed me to discover my cancerous lump—not once but twice. The confidence I had in my body's intuition led me to advocate for myself in the face of Dr. B's mistake. I needed to trust it here, too. I needed to do what made the most sense for me, what made the most sense for my life, and how I wanted to live it.

CHAPTER 27

Members of online breast cancer communities, women to whom this introverted lurker owes so much, said it would be five years post-chemo before I'd feel like myself again. And, as usual, they were right.

Five years after active treatment ended, a sense of a new normalcy crept back into my body, like fauna onto a forest floor after a wildfire. My body was more resilient, my muscles stronger, my brain less muddled. The scars healed and the nerves recovered. Dr. B had told me the skin on my chest would be permanently numb due to nerve damage. But he was wrong. The nerves regenerated and my chest had just as much feeling as before the surgery. What a sweet surprise to feel the soft fuzz of cashmere, the coolness of sheets, and the brush of Mary's hands against my skin.

Out in public, camouflaging my flat chest was no longer a concern. My wardrobe has drifted toward cuts and colors that diminish or flatter a flat chest because they fit me better. My clothes enhance my body's new shape, rather than hide it.

To say my body image has fully recovered would be a lie. But it would also be a lie to infer that my body image was perfect before cancer. With or without breasts, learning to love one's body for all its foibles and flaws is a lifelong process for most people, and I'm content to be perfectly average in this regard. What is true is that seeing my scars in the mirror and baring my flat chest to Mary becomes easier every day, and she has never once suggested I am anything less than beautiful.

Cancer no longer dominates my field of vision, but it casts a long shadow. Rarely does a day go by that breast cancer is not in my line of sight, either because of my occupation or because I've made so many friends who've also dealt with the disease and its aftermath. For my first two years in Massachusetts, I kept doing physical therapy with Cindy, one of the most gifted body workers I'd ever met. She continued to release scar tissue in my chest and nudge my wandering spine back into place. And, of course, I still go every six months to see Dr. P. at the Dana-Farber Cancer Institute in Boston. You can call it the Dana for short.

Get on the Red Line at Davis Square. Ride to Park Street. Transfer to the Green Line. Get off at the Longwood stop and walk four blocks to the Dana. As I push through the glass doors, my face is flushed from walking fast. My legs bound up the lobby stairs two at a time. Waiting for the elevator are doctors with stethoscopes slung around their necks, patients tethered to IV poles, women with bald heads covered by silk scarves, and I am reminded of why I am here. This is a cancer hospital and I am a patient. At the ninth-floor check-in desk, a receptionist secures a white hospital bracelet around my wrist. In the waiting room is my tribe. The women in that room silently but not unkindly check each other out. We look for ourselves. We look for who we hope to be. The woman who gets to the other side, who gets her life back, whose future looks bright.

Dr. P is confident, self-assured, steady. Her capability is without question. She is a lighthouse on which I fix my gaze. She asks me how my writing's going as she palpates my chest wall, then her hands move with assurance to the lymph nodes in my neck and under my arms. The exam is largely performative, but we both play our parts. She the thorough physician, I the patient who has been empowered to make tough choices. Because I've gone off all hormone-lowering drugs, there isn't much for us to discuss about my current situation. I am in a holding pattern. Chances are my body harbors dormant breast cancer cells. We both know sleeper cells are beyond the reach of detection. If my cancer awakens, she won't find it in an office visit. More likely I'll break a bone, develop a chronic cough, or back pain. By then it will have metastasized. We both know that she is on retainer in case this happens.

Reminders of cancer's collateral damage sneak up on me. Three years ago, my left arm became heavy and bloated. The diagnosis was mild lymphedema—without all its lymph nodes, my arm doesn't drain as well as it should and fluid can back up. The old me would have freaked out. Maybe backed away from practicing arm balances in yoga. But post-cancer me took the news in stride and ordered a compression sleeve with a tribal tattoo design. "Love your tats," said a hipster guy in a coffee shop on Boston Common. And, for the rest of the day, I was a compression-sleeve-wearing badass.

On a different day, I stepped out of the sauna at the Boston Sports Club in Davis Square, a towel tightly wrapped around my body. A glimpse at my reflection in the mirror showed my upper chest to be as red as the Citgo sign across the Charles River. The skin that had been radiated is a perfect red square from mid-chest up to clavicle and from mid-sternum around to armpit. Standing outside the gym's sauna, my toes curled against the chilled tile floor. Droplets of sweat clung to the hair at the nape of my neck. I gawked at the red square, evidence of the trauma that lies beneath my surface. A compression sleeve, a radiation burn, an inch-long white scar from a port, these are the nuanced signs of cancer. My flat chest is harder to miss.

One summer day, a stranger at a cafe gives me a knowing look of recognition. I'm wearing a thin, cotton shirt. She sees me, she sees the situation, and she lets me know I've been seen. The look she gives is similar to the glance and nod that passes between queer folks in public spaces. The quick tip of the head, a fleeting acknowledgment, a knowing glance—all are a means of conveying togetherness. A sweet moment of not just witnessing but inclusion that makes my heart swell with love for my people. But I'd never gotten the look from another flat-chested woman. The briefest of eye contact, a nod, an expression that says, "I understand." That day, so accustomed to either passing or being invisible, I am surprised to be seen for who I am and who I chose to be—a woman without breasts, a woman choosing not to hide the body that cancer shaped.

I'd be lying if I said grief did not sneak up on me. The loss of my breasts is most acute during sex. When it's my turn to receive pleasure from Mary, I am self-conscious of what I lack. No more nipples to graze with her hands and lips, no more gentle caressing up top while she works her magic below. It is now Mary who brings the curves to bed. I want to offer her my flat chest with the same openness and generosity she offers me her voluptuousness, but it's not my flat chest she desires so much as my body confidence, which continues to grow.

I prefer the word *remission* to *survivor* because it packs less hubris. For too long, as a journalist, I inadvertently deployed language that obscured the reality of breast cancer, downplayed its seriousness. I'm more careful now. Clarity and truth is what's needed. Language is a good place to start.

Mary is also a stickler for language. The word *marriage* was never one of her favorites. Laden with privilege and patriarchy, the word made her bristle. Even in 2012 when we moved to Massachusetts, where same-sex marriage was legal, she refused to consider marrying me on grounds that she didn't want to exploit a right that queer people in less-progressive states couldn't access. My desire to respect her principles collided head-on with my need to feel like if something happened to me, at least nearby, she'd be able to make decisions about my health care. Burned into my memory was the day Cathy warned us away from the hospital in Martinsville, Indiana, lest Mary be kept from my bedside. Patience is not my strong suit, but luckily I didn't have to wait long. In June 2013, a year after we arrived in New England, the United States Supreme Court struck down DOMA. True to her word, Mary gave in to my desire, and five weeks later on our fifteen-year-dating anniversary, we eloped to Somerville City Hall.

I wore a backless sundress the color of mourning doves. Its halter-style neckline plunged to a deep V in front. Look closely at the photos and you'll see the protrusion of my ribs behind the smooth, soft material. But no one cared, including me.

After we'd finished our vows, the building's fire alarm began to wail. Hesitant to release the moment, the three of us—me, Mary, and the justice of the peace—tried to wait it out, but when Mayor Joe stuck his head in the room and politely asked us to evacuate with everyone else, we gathered our things and headed down the building's main staircase.

A minute later, Mary and I emerged from the front door of Somer-ville City Hall. I held a bouquet of long-stemmed flowers—papery-white lisianthus the size of tea cups, delicate blue nigella, and royal purple verbena. Mary looked dapper in her tailored white shirt and black slacks. Our love was unmistakable. Dozens of City employees who'd been milling around the parking lot, waiting for the all clear from what turned out to be burned toast, began to clap and cheer as we made our way to the sidewalk. She beamed. I blushed. It was perfect in every way. And, in our hastily snapped wedding photos, we are surrounded by two dozen good-natured strangers from our new city, including the Mayor of Somerville and several very handsome firemen. And, in the center of the frame, Mary and I stand side by side, our arms around each other's waists, not wanting to let go. Our smiles as wide open as the sky.

ACKNOWLEDGMENTS

No writer aspires to have material enough for a cancer memoir. A memoir about winning the lottery, yes. Traveling the world in a yacht, absolutely. But cancer? No, thank you. Yet, here I am. But raw material is not enough. I could not have brought this book into the world without the love and support of an incredible group of folks who deserve a world of thanks.

To my dream agent, Helen Zimmermann, thanks for recognizing that I had a story to tell and the persistence to see it through. I will always be grateful for your kindness, good humor, and gentle pointers.

To my editor, Kim Lim, thank you for your attentiveness with my words and your patience with my neurosis.

To my brilliant writing teacher and mentor, Alexandria Marzano-Lesnevich. Thank you for teaching this magazine journalist how to use the tools of fiction to write a literary memoir. The year I spent under your tutelage blew my mind.

Heaps of gratitude to Boston's GrubStreet and the devoted members of the 2014–15 Memoir Incubator cohort: Candace Coakley, Jennifer Duffy, John Hamilton, Ray Matsumiya, Mary Moyer, Andrea Roach, Deborah Schifter, Molly Magram Schpero, and Ann Hardt Williams. Each of you read early drafts of this book at least three times, and your kind, gentle, insightful feedback helped me bring my story to life.

Thank you to my generous and effusive beta readers: Howard Axelrod, Krista Bremer, Kim Kopetz-Buttleman, Susan Gubar, Mary

Jane Minkin, Bonnie Mioduchoski, Angela Palm, Mike Scalise, Robin Schoenthaler, Suzanna Walters, and Florence Williams. Your words of encouragement kept me going through some tough times.

Special thanks to my dazzling graphic designer, Teresita Obra Olson, and my last-push cheerleading squad: Christie Aschwanden, Kelly Ford, Beth Grossman, and Jennifer Lunden.

My heart is full of gratitude for my beloved Bloomington friends and my Facebook tribes, including Flat & Fabulous, Breastless & Beautiful, and QueerCancer. Thank you for providing space for flatties and unis to build community.

My writing evolved thanks to wonderful people I met at Bread Loaf Writers' Conference and the Vermont Studio Center. And a book award from the Kentucky Women Writers Conference was a meaningful acknowledgment of my work in progress.

Special thanks to the team of body workers who help make my body habitable: Tom Alden, Dell Fisher, Ramona Leeman, Mariann Sisco, Patricia Stepan, and Kay Thorbecke. Thanks, too, to Fez Aswat, Nicoline Valkenberg, and the teachers at Samara Yoga who welcomed my cranky, fidgety, resistant-to-group-instruction self into class several times a week. And thank you to the staff of Somerville's Diesel Cafe and 3 Little Figs for keeping me caffeinated.

To dear Emma, the best and brattiest dog ever, who died during the writing of this book. She was my sidekick for thirteen years, and my side will never be the same.

I would like to remember my friend Cindy Cardillo who was diagnosed with breast cancer and died of the disease shortly thereafter. She was a gifted healer, and she is deeply missed.

To my family, no one is thrilled to find a memoirist in their midst but you have been heroically supportive and patient. You've encouraged me to follow my writer bliss, even when it meant writing about you—and not always casting you in your best light—and for that shot of realness I am grateful.

Finally, to Mary, my partner in all things. If you haven't noticed, this book is one long love letter to you. None of this would have been possible without your unflagging support. Never (not even once) in my five years of total preoccupation with this project did you indicate a shred of doubt that I would succeed. You believe in me more than I believe in myself. Your unstoppable energy and optimism have buoyed me through life and carried me to places I never could have imagined. Sharing my days with someone as insightful, articulate, reflective, and brilliant as you is like having hitched my wagon to a shooting star. Plus, you are sexy as hell. It is both a coincidence and not that the publishing of this book coincides with our twentieth anniversary. You are my constant.